Child Spacing and Reproductive Health in Rural Karnataka, India

From Research to Action

INGE HUTTER, N.V. RAJESWARI,
J.S. HALLAD AND B.M. RAMESH

IDPAD

MANOHAR
2006

First published December 2006

ISBN 81-7304-714-6

Published by

Ajay Kumar Jain for
Manohar Publishers & Distributors
4753/23 Ansari Road, Daryaganj
New Delhi 110 002

Typeset at

Digigrafics
New Delhi 110 049

Printed at

Lordson Publishers Pvt. Ltd.
Delhi 110 007

Distributed in South Asia by

FOUNDATION BOOKS

4381/4, Ansari Road
Daryaganj, New Delhi 110 002
and its branches at Mumbai, Hyderabad,
Bangalore, Chennai, Kolkata

Contents

Preface

This book presents and discusses the research project 'Reproductive Health and Child Spacing in Rural Karnataka', conducted by the Population Research Centre, Faculty of Spatial Sciences of the University of Groningen, and the Population Research Centre, Institute of Economic Research in Dharwad, and it is based on earlier interim reports (Hutter 1998; Rajeswari and Hutter 1998; Hutter, Rajeswari, Hallad and Ramesh 1999; Hutter, Ramesh, Rajarama and Riiti 2002).

We are thankful to IDPAD (Indo-Dutch Programme on Alternatives in Development) in The Hague (Dr. Marc Verhagen; Dr. Cora Govers) and ICSSR (Indian Council of Social Science Research) in Delhi (Ms. Sanchita Dutta) for the funding of our research.

The research project was conducted in the period 1996-2000 in 11 villages of Dharwad *taluka* in Dharwad district of Karnataka. From the very beginning, the objective was to conduct academic research but also to ensure that research findings would be used to benefit the research subjects and improve the reproductive health status of women and men in the villages in Dharwad *taluka*. The research project thus was followed up with an evidence-based educational intervention called Spandana, a collaboration of the two research institutes with the Family Planning Association of India (FPAI), Dharwad branch. Spandana has been implemented in villages around Dharwad (in 2006 the programme reached more than 30 villages) during the period 2000-6.

Chapter 10 of this book, on research-for-action, is co-authored with S.V. Morab, S.V. Kulkarni and Sujata F. Panigatti from FPAI, Dharwad/Spandana. This chapter concerns the first phase of Spandana (2000-2003).

We gratefully acknowledge IDPAD in The Hague / ICSSR in Delhi for their keen interest in the translation of our IDPAD research into action and the funding provided for part of this exercise. Marc Verhagen, then Coordinator of IDPAD, deserves

special thanks, not only for the IDPAD funding but also for being instrumental in our contacts with the Bernard van Leer Foundation, which subsequently funded Spandana for six years. Special thanks go to Liana Gertsch and Jeannet van de Korput of the Bernard van Leer Foundation for their always stimulating, critical and reflective discussions on Spandana.

Furthermore, the authors wish to thank Dr. P.N. Mari Bhat, Director of PRC Dharwad where fieldwork was conducted in 1996-7; Dr. T. Rajaretnam, Deputy Director of PRC Dharwad; Prof. Frans Willekens, former Head of Department of PRC Groningen; and acknowledge the collaborative research programme HERA of PRC Groningen and NIDI (Netherlands Interdisciplinary Demographic Institute) in The Hague. The authors are indebted to all research and supportive faculty at PRC Dharwad for valuable suggestions, their efforts and strong support during the fieldwork; to all ad-hoc research staff appointed for the project; and to village leaders, influential persons and key informants in the villages for their support. Our thanks also to Gina Rozario for editing the English language of manuscript, and bringing attention to the expressions used in the transcripts of in-depth interviews conducted in the local language Kannada and their subsequent translation into English.

Last, but definitely not least, we gratefully acknowledge the women and men in the villages around Dharwad where we conducted our research: for receiving us with genuine warm hospitality in their homes; for their willingness to talk about reproductive health and sensitive issues such as sexuality; and inviting us to participate in certain events in their lives (e.g. Hooli in T. Ramachandra Nagar; several wedding ceremonies in Mavinkoppa).

We hope we have done justice to their questions at the time of our research, namely how this research could and would help you? Through Spandana we hope to have kept our promise, which was to present and use the research results for their benefit and to improve the reproductive health status of both women and men in Dharwad *taluka*.

Dharwad
18 August 2006

INGE HUTTER, N.V. RAJESWARI,
JYOTHI S. HALLAD AND B.M. RAMESH

1

Introduction

The survival of both women and children is negatively related to childbearing at the fringes of the reproductive period (under 18 and over 35 years of age), to high parity (4+) and short birth intervals (less than 24 months). Child spacing is an important factor that can contribute to healthier children and improve their chances of survival. Chances of survival of children born after a birth interval of one year or less, for example, are half or even less than that for children born after an interval of two years or more (Kusum, 1983; WHO, 1984, Isaacs and Fincancioglu, 1989, Hobcraft et al., 1985). Similar results, i.e. higher survival chances for children born after a longer birth interval, have been confirmed for India (Nath et al., 1994, Gujral et al., 1992, Dhanalakshmi, 1993; Bhargava et al., 1991; Kost and Amin, 1992). The effects of child spacing on the health status of women, however, are far less researched and documented.

A short birth interval, i.e. less than 24 months, is one of the factors indicating a pregnancy at risk (WHO, 1991). Lack of adequate spacing between pregnancies increases the risks to the mother as she does not have enough time to recover from the added physical demands made upon her by pregnancy and lactation (Population Reference Bureau, 1986; WHO, 1991; DGIS, 1994). In other words, a short birth interval is related to the so-called 'maternal depletion syndrome', indicated by Chronic Energy Deficiency (CED) (see James et al., 1988; Kusin et al., 1992; 1994a, b) and Body Mass Index (BMI) (weight/height[1]).

Earlier research in the area of Dharwad *taluka* in Karnataka, India, on women's nutrition during pregnancy and the birth weight of their children (Hutter, 1994) indicated that the majority (62 per cent) of women were chronically malnourished (BMI

below 18.5) even before they became pregnant. Moreover, almost half of the women had pregnancy outcome intervals of less than 24 months. Results from the Indian National Family Health Survey (NFHS) (1998-9), the Demographic Health Survey (DHS) Nepal (2001) and DHS Bangladesh (2004) indicate lower percentages of women whose BMI was below 18.5: 41 per cent, 27 per cent and 38 per cent, respectively (www.measuredhs.com).

This book[2] focuses on child spacing behaviour studied from a reproductive health perspective. Following the International Conference on Population and Development (ICPD) of 1994 in Cairo, child spacing has become one of the elements constituting the reproductive health career of women. Child spacing is thus related to other reproductive health events in a woman's life—first menstruation, marriage and pregnancy histories including abortions—and to reproductive health processes such as menstruation, gynaecological morbidity, perceived reproductive health status, malnutrition and sexuality. In addition, a reproductive health approach to child spacing entails paying due attention to people's needs, choices and ambitions, and their reproductive rights.

The following research questions are central in the book:

1. What is the actual child spacing behaviour of women and its proximate determinants (Bongaarts and Potter, 1983) as situated in
   - the life course, i.e. situating child spacing behaviour in relation to other reproductive health events and processes in the reproductive career?
2. What are the women's and men's perceptions and the accompanying decision-making processes they undergo regarding child spacing and other reproductive health events and processes in the life course; what are their motivations for behaviour; perceptions and beliefs; decision-making processes; cultural schemas on health, relationships, and children as situated in
   - a changing economic, social and cultural context?
   - a gender context, where the status of women undergoes changes over the life course?

The theoretical framework includes the model of Bongaarts

and Potter (1983) and Becker (1993) and the process-context approach as formulated by Willekens (1990; 1992), De Bruijn (1992; 1993; 1999), Hutter (1998) (see Chapter 2).

Fieldwork was conducted in the period 1996-9, and it adopted a multi-level research methodology, involving both quantitative and qualitative research. The quantitative methods of census and survey provide information on actual child spacing behaviour within the reproductive career. The qualitative methods of in-depth interviews obtained the views of women and men about their spacing and reproductive health behaviour. A census was conducted in the 11 research villages in Dharwad *taluka*. From there, women were selected as respondents for participation in a survey from which they were selected for in-depth interviews. In-depth interviews among men were conducted in one of the research villages. The methodology of the research is further described in Chapter 3.

The census data provides the socio-economic and demographic contexts of the villages in which child spacing and reproductive health behaviour was studied. The census data collected in 1996 provides a continuity with the census data collected in the same villages in 1991, enabling us to identify changes that occurred in the research area over five years. For a description of the research area and study population, see Chapter 4.

Actual child spacing behaviour within the reproductive career is described in Chapter 5, while perceptions and beliefs of women and men regarding fertility and birth intervals are reported in Chapter 6. Results on decision-making processes, perceptions and cultural schemas on contraceptive use are elaborated in Chapter 7. Major reasons for not using spacing methods are perceived negative health effects. In addition, the weakness syndrome turns out to be a major underlying factor. The cultural schemas, embedded in the cultural meaning system at large, underlying child spacing and reproductive health are subsequently described in Chapter 8. Among these schemas, especially those on 'heating and cooling' and 'purity and pollution' play an important role.

Another major reason for not using spacing methods, as women in the reproductive ages indicate, is the perceived social influence of others in the environment, especially husbands and

mothers-in-law. The decision-making power and status of women as it changes over the life course is described in Chapter 9. Status and decision-making power change with transitions from one life stage to another, for example, a transition from not having reached menarche to having reached menarche or from not being married to married. We not only inquire about the personal experiences of women, but also about (expected) changes in behaviour, feelings and emotions during these different transitions.

The research aims at contributing scientific evidence for interventions and programmes to improve the reproductive health status of women. Results of the research therefore have been translated in the reproductive health intervention programme Spandana[3] which is a collaboration between the authors and the NGO Family Planning Association of India (FPAI), Dharwad Branch. Chapter 10 describes how the research results are translated into intervention, taking into account actual behaviour, needs, perceptions, socio-economic circumstances and the cultural meaning attached to reproductive health events.

NOTES

1. 'Reproductive Health and Child Spacing in Rural Karnataka, India' was a research collaboration between the Population Research Centre (PRC), University of Groningen, The Netherlands, and the Population Research Centre, J.S.S. Institute of Economic Research (IER), Dharwad, Karnataka, India.
   The project was funded by IDPAD (Indo-Dutch Programme on Alternatives in Development), The Hague, and ICSSR (Indian Council of Social Science Research), New Delhi.
2. The book is based on earlier interim reports. For more information, please see the background report on the project (Hutter, 1998), the basic census report (Rajeswari and Hutter, 1998), the basic survey report (Hutter, Rajeswari, Hallad and Ramesh, 1999) and the basic report comprising in-depth interviews and female and male perspectives (Hutter, Ramesh, Rajarama and Riiti, 2002).
3. Funded by the Bernard van Leer Foundation, The Hague, and partly by IDPAD.

2

Theoretical Framework on Child Spacing Behaviour and Decision-making

The following research questions were presented in the introduction:

1. What is the actual child spacing behaviour of women and its proximate determinants as situated in
   - the life course, i.e. situating child spacing behaviour in relation to other reproductive health events and processes in the reproductive career?
2. What are the women's and men's perceptions and accompanying decision-making processes they undergo regarding child spacing; what are their motivations for behaviour; perceptions and beliefs; decision-making processes; cultural schemas on health, relationships, and children as situated in
   - a changing economic, social and cultural context?
   - a gender context, where the status of women undergoes changes over the life course?

Next, we discuss the models and theoretical frameworks that inform the research.

Overall, a life course approach is adopted, i.e. present child spacing behaviour is seen as the outcome of past behaviour and which will influence future behaviour. Thus, child spacing behaviour is situated within the reproductive health career of women (Section 2.1), starting with menarche (Section 2.1.1) and ending with sterility or menopause (Section 2.1.2). Child spacing behaviour, indicated by the length of birth intervals and their

biological and behavioural determinants, is analysed with the aid of models developed by Bongaarts and Potter (1983) and Becker (1993) (Sections 2.1.3 and 2.1.4).

Child spacing and reproductive health behaviour are viewed as the outcome of decision-making processes that take place within the context in which people live, the so-called process-context approach (see Willekens, 1990 and 1992; De Bruijn, 1992, 1993 and 1999; Hutter, 1998). Theories on motivation of behaviour, the model proposed by Ajzen and Fishbein (1980) and Ajzen (1991) (cultural) schemas motivating behaviour (D'Andrade, 1984 and 1995) guide the research on decision-making processes entailed in child spacing behaviour (Section 2.2).

2.1 The Life Course: Child Spacing Behaviour within the Reproductive Career

In the research, we adopt a life course perspective: former experiences, expectations and circumstances in earlier stages of the life course determine what people do at present [Erikson (1980) cited by Willekens, 1989; Greenhalgh, 1994; Carter (1996) cited by Greenhalgh, 1995]. The life course can be defined as 'the sequence of events and experiences in a life from birth until death and the chain of personal states and encountered situations which influence and are influenced by this sequence of events' (Runyan, 1984: 82). Within the life course, life events occur.

From the life course perspective, women follow a particular reproductive health career. A career is 'the chain of stable and transition periods pertaining to a given domain' (Willekens, 1989: 8). A career is 'a route to goal achieveme It is, therefore, not only a sequence of events and stages, but it is a goal directed or purposive sequence.' Careers can be associated with each attribute or characteristic of a person that changes over a lifetime (Willekens, 1989). The reproductive health career of women for example is closely intertwined with their educational career, job career, and marriage and family building career.

The reproductive health career of women starts with the event of menarche, followed by life events such as marriage or more

relevantly the start of sexual relationships, pregnancies, outcomes of those pregnancies (live birth, still birth, spontaneous abortion, induced abortion), menopause or sterilization. Life events are universal, i.e. they happen in all societies. However, the timing and meaning of these events are influenced by the context in which people live. Celebration of the events in a society, for example, the so-called *rite de passage*, is conducted in a way that is particular and significant to that society.

Bongaarts and Potter (1983), in examining various events which directly influence the duration of the reproductive career, derived a set of proximate determinants from earlier formulated immediate determinants of fertility (Davis and Blake, 1956). The most important characteristic of a proximate determinant is 'its direct influence on fertility' (Bongaarts and Potter, 1983: 1-2). The potential reproductive period starts with menarche, and Bongaarts and Potter (1983) state that in most societies socially sanctioned childbearing is accorded to women in relatively stable sexual relationships. They use the term marriage, but actually mean the start of sexual relationships. Marriage or sexual union thus in practice is commonly taken as the starting point of the reproductive career. Once married or in a sexual relationship, a woman is considered to be at risk of childbearing until she is permanently sterile or menopausal, unless her career is interrupted by a divorce, separation or widowhood. While married and fecund, women reproduce at a rate that is inversely related to the average duration of the birth interval (Bongaarts and Potter, 1983).

Bongaarts and Potter (1983) subsequently identify the proximate determinants and duration of birth intervals as constituted by postpartum infecundability, waiting time to conception and nine months of pregnancy. Intra-uterine mortality (spontaneous abortion, stillbirth or induced abortion) extends the length of a birth interval. Postpartum infecundability is constituted by postpartum amenorrhoea due to breastfeeding and postpartum abstinence. The duration of waiting time to conception is determined by the rate of conception, which in turn is related to frequency of sexual intercourse and the level and effectiveness of contraceptive use (Bongaarts and Potter, 1983: 29-30).

This research focuses on child spacing behaviour, i.e. the duration of birth intervals and proximate determinants such as postpartum amenorrhoea, breastfeeding, postpartum abstinence, abortions, stillbirths, and contraceptive use. Child spacing behaviour is situated in the reproductive career, starting with menarche and consummation of marriage and ending in menopause or sterilisation. In India, the latter is a more common practice.

The model of Bongaarts and Potter (1983) focuses on events in the reproductive career rather than the reproductive *health* career. Underlying factors and reproductive health indicators such as gynaecological morbidity, sexuality, malnutrition, menstruation, and reproductive health issues that might occur after menopause are excluded from their model. Sexuality underlies the whole reproductive career and rules and perceptions regarding menstruation, the monthly reproductive cycle of women. Malnutrition might affect not only age at menarche (Bosch, 2005), but also lead to sub-fecundity in women which in turn could affect the duration of birth interval (Ford and Huffman, 1993). Gynaecological morbidity might affect the duration of birth intervals (Rahman and Menken, 1993; Baird et al., 1993; Cates et al., 1993).

In the following sections, we examine the literature on the different events in the reproductive career and proximate determinants of birth intervals. The literature will help us to interpret the results of the research presented especially in Chapter 5 on child spacing behaviour. Most of the information is derived from Bongaarts and Potters (1983) and Gray and Spira (1993).

2.1.1 MENARCHE

Becker (1993) provides an extensive review of studies on median ages at menarche. The difference between the highest and lowest age at menarche is about four years. Differences between industrialized and developing countries are evident. New Guinea, Rwanda, the Philippines and rural populations show the highest ages (between 17-18 years), Western and urban populations the

lowest ages (around 12.4 years). Over the last decades, age at menarche in general is decreasing. In 1840, age at menarche in industrialized countries was 16.5 years, at present it is around 13 years. The trend of declining age at menarche, however, seems to be levelling off (Rees, 1995).

The reasons behind the declining age at menarche are not completely clear. Different authors mention different, but more or less related factors. Rees (1995) identifies the improvement in health and environmental conditions; Bongaarts and Potter (1983) attribute it to an increase in body size and improved diet; for Becker (1993) it was improved nutritional status and socio-economic circumstances; Riley et al. (1993) found nutritional status, in particular weight to be important while Bosch (2005) highlights the nutritional status during adolescence and childhood, in particular stunting. The most commonly mentioned factor thus is nutritional status. Several studies, conducted in the USA and India, indicate a direct relationship between food intake/ nutritional status and menarche [Dreizen et al. (1967) and Bhalla and Shrivata (1974) cited by Riley et al. 1993]. In Matlab, Bangladesh, age at menarche increased from 12.9 years in 1961 to 17.4 years in 1977 which is ascribed to the declining nutritional conditions during the 1971 war and 1974 famine [Chowdhury et al. (1977) cited by Becker, 1993].

Another factor influencing age at menarche is rigorous exercise: athletes and ballet dancers experience menarche at a later age, due to lower body weight and less body fat (Cumming, 1993). It is not clear whether activities conducted by girls in developing countries, for example, fetching water, carrying wood, agricultural activities, might affect their age at menarche (Riley et al., 1993).

In which way can age at menarche affect fertility of women? A lower age at menarche implies lengthening of the potential reproductive period. That is, in principle, women can have more children during their lifetime. However, after menarche adolescent sub-fecundity and foetal wastage can play a role (Riley et al., 1993). Also, declining ages at menarche generally go hand in hand with increasing ages at marriage, thus shortening the potential reproductive period (Bongaarts and Potter, 1983).

Several studies indicate a strong correlation between age at menarche and age at marriage (Udry and Cliquet, 1982; Sandler et al. (1984) cited by Riley, 1993).

Results of studies on adolescent sub-fecundity are not unanimous. Anovulatory and aluteal cycles are reported to occur more frequently immediately after menarche, but ovulatory cycles also take place. A few studies in developing countries report long periods of adolescent sub-fecundity. Nair (1983) claims that Indian adolescent sub-fertility lasts up to the age of 19 or 20 years. For Bangladeshi women, Foster et al. (1986) conclude that the period of adolescent sterility was significantly shorter among women who had their menarche at a higher age. Studies in industrialized countries, however, indicate a reverse relation: late age at menarche was related to a longer period of adolescent sub-fertility (Riley et al., 1993).

2.1.2 PERMANENT STERILITY OR MENOPAUSE

The median age at menopause, defined as the cessation of menstruation, is reported to be 50 years among Caucasian women (Rahman and Menken, 1993). Gray (1979, cited by Rahman and Menken, 1993) mentioned more variation among non-Caucasian women: among Punjabi women (India) menopause occurs at 43.4 years, among Bantu women (South Africa) it is 49.7 years. The same author predicted that the likelihood of permanent sterility at age 35 is less than 20 per cent, at age 40 about 40 per cent, and at age 45 about 80 per cent (cited by Jansen, 1984).

A couple of studies, conducted in the USA, Bangladesh and New Guinea, reported that women with less weight experienced a lower age at menopause. Jansen (1984) reported that poor nutrition in India appears to lower the age at menopause. However, McKinlay (1985, cited by Rahman and Menken, 1993) mentions the relationship between nutrition and age at menopause to be insignificant. A statistical significant relationship was found only between age at menopause and smoking: smokers tend to reach menopause earlier than non-smokers.

Throughout the reproductive period fecundity gradually declines. Age-specific marital fertility rates among natural

fertility populations, as indicated by Coale and Trussel (1974), show declines from age group 20-4 onwards with accelerated faster declines after age 35 (see Table 2.1).

TABLE 2.1: STANDARD SCHEDULE OF NATURAL MARITAL FERTILITY

Age group (years)	*Relative Marital Fertility*
20-4	100
25-9	94
30-4	86
35-9	70
40-4	36
40-5	5

Source: Coale and Trussel, 1974.

Two measurements are commonly used to indicate the end of the reproductive career: the mean age at last birth and the age-specific prevalence of sterility or infecundity (the physiological incapacity to produce a live birth). Among natural fertility populations, the mean age at birth of the last child would approximately be the age at onset of sterility (Rahman and Menken, 1993). Knodel (1978) estimated this mean age to be around 40 years.

Using historical data from seventeenth- and eighteenth-century France and early twentieth-century Hutterites, Bongaarts (1982, cited by Rahman and Menken 1993) estimated age-specific sterility levels (see Table 2.2).

TABLE 2.2: AGE-SPECIFIC STERILITY: PROPORTION OF WOMEN STERILE BY AGE FOR SEVENTEENTH- AND EIGHTEENTH-CENTURY FRANCE AND TWENTIETH-CENTURY HUTTERITES

Age group	%	
(years)	*France*	*Hutterites*
20-4	5	3
25-9	6	3
30-4	10	9
35-9	18	22

Source: Bongaarts, 1982.

Rahman and Menken (1993) compared these figures with data from the World Fertility Survey (WFS). A woman was considered to be in-fecund when she reported to be unable to conceive, or if she did not have a child during the last five years prior to the survey and had not used contraception in that period. The WFS data show much higher figures for the older age groups than Bongaarts' (1982) estimations. Among women aged 20-24, the highest percentage of in-fecundity was found in Nepal (9 per cent), Bangladesh (8 per cent), Haiti and Trinidad and Tobago (7 per cent both). Among women aged 25-29, the highest percentages were found in Lesotho (16 per cent), Sudan, Indonesia, Costa Rica and Jamaica (13 per cent, all). Among women aged 35-39, the highest percentages were found in Indonesia (51 per cent), Costa Rica (48 per cent), Guyana (46 per cent), Sudan and Trinidad and Tobago (44 per cent). These figures seem to be high and one might question whether indeed in-fecundity is being measured here or whether it is infertility, i.e. not realised fertility which might be affected by traditional customs such as abstinence.

Low fertility prior to menopause is related to both biological and socio-cultural factors (Rahman and Menken, 1993). With increasing age, fecundability (capacity to conceive) declines while spontaneous foetal wastage increases. In addition, sterility and higher foetal loss can be related to sexually transmitted diseases (STDs), malaria, obstetric and genital tract traumas, and postpartum sepsis (Rahman and Menken, 1993: 81-2). STDs induce tubal infertility, thus reducing fecundability (Baird, et al., 1993), predominantly through Pelvic Inflammatory Disease (PID). Key organisms involved are gonorrhoea, chlamydia trachomatis and anaerobic bacteria frequently associated with bacterial vaginosis (Cates et al., 1993: 116).

Weinstein et al. (1993: 225) claim that fecundability is heterogeneous within populations. The authors suggest that this heterogeneity has a biological source: differences among women in the level of intra-uterine mortality, incidence of anovulatory cycles, as well as in total cycle length.

Socio-cultural factors related to low fertility in the period preceding menopause are coital frequency and terminal abstinence. Frequency of intercourse is generally believed to

decline with age. In addition, some societies do follow explicit rules that indicate the end of sexual relationships, such as the 'grandmother complex' in India.

2.1.3 WAITING TIME TO CONCEPTION AND FECUNDABILITY: BECKER'S MODEL (1993)

Bongaarts and Potter (1983: 29-30) link waiting time to conception to rate of conception. According to them, the most widely used measure of conception rate is fecundability, i.e. the probability of conceiving in a month among fecund women—disregarding pregnant, sterile and amenorrhoeic women. Fecundability is inversely related to the duration of waiting time to conception. A typical of value of fecundability for non-contracepting women is 0.2. That means, in a group of fecund women 20 per cent can be expected to conceive in the first month of exposure to the risk of conception.

Becker (1993), based on James (1979) and Bongaarts and Potter (1983), presents a model of the reproductive process in which he estimates recognized fecundability (F), i.e. the probability that a recognizable conception occurs during a menstrual cycle. The model gives a good insight into the different stages preceding conception and birth, and related background factors. As this is highly useful and relevant to our research (see Chapter 5), we reproduce the model briefly here. According to Becker (1993) recognized fecundability depends on:

p_1 = the probability that a menstrual cycle is ovulatory;

p_2 = the probability that insemination takes place (coitus) during the fertile period given that ovulation occurs;

p_3 = the probability that insemination leads to fertilization given that it occurs during the fertile period; and

p_4 = the probability that conception is recognizable given that fertilization occurs.

To distinguish pregnancies that result in live births Becker (1993) defines F′ which is the probability that a live birth conception occurs during a menstrual cycle. F′ is estimated as $F \times p_5$, where:

p_5 = the probability of a live birth given that conception is recognized (Becker 1993: 29).

The first factor (the probability that a menstrual cycle is ovulatory) and the fourth factor (the probability that conception is recognizable given that fertilization occurs) are both biological in character. The second, the third, and the fifth factors are also determined by human behaviour. The probability of insemination during the fertile period (p_2), for example, is affected by the timing and the frequency of intercourse. The probability that insemination leads to fertilization (p_3) depends on the use of contraceptive methods. The probability of a live birth once conception has taken place (p_5) depends on whether an abortion is induced or not.

In the following sections, we briefly discuss the five different factors identified by Becker (1993) and others.

(i) Probability that a Menstrual Cycle is Ovulatory

Several studies indicate that the percentage of ovulatory cycles is low right after menarche, then increases slowly and reaches a maximum in the mid- and late 1920s. Results from a German study show the decreasing trend in anovular cycles, changing from 60 per cent among women aged 12-14, to 43 per cent among women aged 15-17, to 13 per cent among for women aged 21-25 and 5 per cent among women aged 26-30 years (Doring, 1969, cited by Becker, 1993).

In general, fecundability is higher when cycles are regular (Spira et al., 1993). Ovarian cycle length varies with age: they are longer and more variable right after menarche and before menopause (Weinstein et al., 1993: 210). In Bangladesh, a greater variability in length of cycles was found (Menken, 1975, cited by Becker, 1993). Also, an Indian study indicated higher variability in cycle length in the period following menarche and before menopause (Jeyaseelan and Antonisamy, 1992). The last-mentioned authors contend that the 28 days norm is not applicable to developing countries.

(ii) Probability of Coitus in the Fertile Period: Frequency of Intercourse

In most societies, sexual relationships are allowed within socially approved relationships, i.e. within marriage. Age at marriage and

proportion of women married is an important determinant of (adolescent) fertility. Frequency of intercourse has been studied in only a few countries. The first part of Table 2.3 provides data on the frequency of intercourse in a four-week period for women younger than 20 years and between 20-24 years in Bangladesh and India. Frequency of intercourse in the first group was around 9 to 10 times per cycle of 4 weeks. In the second group, frequency varied between 6 to almost 10 times per cycle of 4 weeks. In general, coital frequency declines with age and marital duration (Rahman and Menken, 1993; Udry, 1993; Becker, 1993).

A more recent study in rural Bangladesh by Islam and Khan (1993) reports a strong decline in coital frequency with age. A study in Taiwan (1986) reports a similar decline by age, but with much lower frequencies: from 5.1 among women aged 20-24 years to 2.2 among women aged 45-49 years (Weinstein et al., 1993). The latter authors rightly conclude that besides frequency of intercourse, the timing of intercourse within the cycle is an important behavioural determinant of fecundability (Weinstein et al., 1993).

An interesting feature in the study by Islam and Khan (1993) in rural Bangladesh is the information on frequency of intercourse

TABLE 2.3: FREQUENCY OF INTERCOURSE FOR WOMEN IN DIFFERENT AGE CATEGORIES, IN A FOUR-WEEK PERIOD (BANGLADESH, INDIA), DURING THE LAST MONTH (BANGLADESH AND TAIWAN).

Country	*Age*						
	< 20	*20-4*					
Bangladesh (1978)[a]	9.2	6.8					
India, Bombay (1970-9)[b]	10.0	9.6					
				Age			
	15-19	*20-4*	*25-9*	*30-4*	*35-9*	*40-4*	*45-9*
Bangladesh (1988-9)[c]	10.8	10.2	8.7	6.9	5.5	4.5	3.7
Taiwan (1986)[d]	5.1	4.5	4.1	3.6	2.8	2.2	

Sources: a. Ruzicka and Bhatia, 1982;
b. Kapoor and Aravindakshan, 1980;
c. Weinstein et al., 1993;
d. Islam and Khan, 1993.

among different socio-economic groups. Hindus, for example, appeared to have higher frequencies of intercourse than Muslims. However, this contradicts the research by Nag (1972, cited by Islam and Khan, 1993) who found higher frequencies of intercourse among Muslims in India. In addition, in Bangladesh the frequency of intercourse increased with higher educational levels. One might wonder whether this finding does really reflect frequency of intercourse or the fact that educated respondents might be more forthcoming about frequency of intercourse. Moreover, women living in nuclear families reported higher frequencies of intercourse than women who lived in joint families. However, it is clear that measurement of frequency of intercourse remains a difficult issue.

Bongaarts and Potter's (1983: 29-30) model estimates of fecundability and conception wait for different coital rates are presented in Table 2.4. A frequency of intercourse of 10 times per menstrual cycle means a fecundability of 0.284 and a waiting

TABLE 2.4: MODEL ESTIMATES OF FECUNDABILITY AND CONCEPTION WAIT FOR DIFFERENT COITAL RATES

Number of Coitus per Menstrual Cycle	*Fecundability*	*Approx. Duration of Conception Wait (months)*
1	0.035	42.8
2	0.068	22.1
3	0.100	15.0
4	0.130	11.5
5	0.159	9.4
6	0.187	8.0
7	0.213	7.0
8	0.238	6.3
9	0.262	5.7
10	0.284	5.3
11	0.305	4.9
12	0.324	4.6
13	0.342	4.4
14	0.359	4.2
15	0.374	4.0
20	0.429	3.5

Source: Bongaarts and Potter, 1983: 34.

time to conception of approximately 5.3 months. A frequency of 20 times per cycle means fecundability of 0.429 and a waiting time to conception of only 3.5 months (Bongaarts and Potter, 1983).

Besides age and marriage duration, studies have identified other factors related to the frequency of intercourse. The use of the pill has been mentioned as a factor increasing the frequency of intercourse (Westhoff et al., 1969). Udry (1993) mentions trends of coitus taking place on specific days, such as the weekends in the USA. Of course, frequency of intercourse also depends on the presence of both spouses, housing or sleeping facilities and cultural rules on abstinence (discussed later).

(iii) Probability of Fertilization Given Coitus in the Fertile Period: The Contraceptive Prevalence Rate

As mentioned before, frequency of intercourse is not the only factor determining the probability of conception; the timing of intercourse is also highly important. For women having intercourse within 24 hours of the time of ovulation, the probability of conception, given that coitus takes place and that no contraceptives are used, has been estimated to be 0.85 (Hertig, 1967). Bongaarts and Potter (1983) regard this an underestimation and according to their calculation it is 0.95.

As mentioned before, the probability of fertilization is mainly determined by the level and the effectiveness of contraceptive use (p_3 is estimated as the sum of the various contraceptive methods). The Contraceptive Prevalence Rate (CPR), i.e. the percentage of married women in the reproductive period currently using a contraceptive, is the result of new acceptors and continuing and discontinuing users.

(iv) Probability a Conception is Recognized Given Fertility Occurs: Early Foetal Loss

Most reproductive loss occurs before a pregnancy is even detected (Baird et al., 1993: 333). Hertig (1967) estimated that the probability of recognition of a conception is 0.5, i.e. half of all fertilized ova abort before the conception is realized (cited by

Bongaarts and Potter, 1983: 33; Becker, 1993: 38). Early foetal loss will probably not be detected, or it may be viewed as delayed menstruation.

Wilcox et al. (1993) observed that 22 per cent of embryos are aborted between implantation and recognition of pregnancy. Including spontaneous abortions, the total loss was 32 per cent. Based on these data, the authors estimate the proportion of fertilized embryos which abort between fertilization and implantation to be 0.39. In his application of the model for the USA, Becker estimated the probability that a conception is recognized to be 60 per cent.

Simpson and Carson (1993) estimated that of all recognized pregnancies 10 to 15 per cent are lost during the first trimester, while an additional 2 to 3 per cent are lost later in pregnancy, and many more conceptions are lost without any recognition. The authors describe several factors associated with early foetal loss such as chromosomal abnormalities, diabetes mellitus, intra-uterine surgery, but also infections, smoking, alcohol, environmental chemicals, maternal morbidity, traumas, IUDs and other contraceptives (see Simpson and Carson, 1993).

(v) Probability of Live Birth Given that Conception is Recognized: Spontaneous Abortions, Stillbirths and Induced Abortion

Spontaneous abortions are defined (WHO, 1991) as the termination of pregnancy before 28 weeks of gestation. Pregnancy losses at 28 weeks or later are classified as stillbirths. The probability of spontaneous abortion is generally recognized as being biologically determined. Singh and Wulf (1994: 12) estimate that spontaneous abortions between 17 and 27 weeks of pregnancy constitute 2.48 per cent of all live births. Wilcox et al. (1985, cited by Becker, 1993) estimate 4 losses in 17 pregnancies.

In the former 1991-2 research in Karnataka (Hutter, 1994) a group of 186 women was followed throughout pregnancy, from the stage of pre-pregnancy onwards. The study indicated that 12.3 per cent of all pregnant women had a spontaneous abortion. Another 5.9 per cent of all pregnancies ended in stillbirth. Most of these stillbirths (N = 8) were macerated stillbirths. Three were

fresh stillbirths, i.e. children who died during the process of labour.

The incidence of induced abortion is difficult to estimate: illegal, not registered abortions form a considerable proportion of all induced abortions. The International Planned Parenthood Federation (IPPF) estimates that worldwide between one-fifth and one-third of all pregnancies are terminated by induced abortions (IPPF, 1993: 23).

It is generally agreed that very young women are at an increased risk of spontaneous abortions (Roman and Stevenson (1983) cited by Becker, 1993). Weinstein et al. (1993), reviewing nine studies, found the following age pattern for early foetal loss. Among women aged 20-24 the probability of early foetal loss is 0.3. The probability then declines and starts to increase again from the late 1920s onwards. Simpson and Carson (1993) state that women aged 40-44 experience approximately twice the likelihood of a foetal loss (Simpson and Carson, 1993: 307-8). In former times, women who experienced more than three spontaneous abortions were classified as so-called 'habitual aborters'. Simpson and Carson (1993: 308), however, conclude that among women with at least one live birth the recurrence risk of spontaneous abortion is 25-30 per cent, while among women with no live birth the risk is higher at 40 per cent.

2.1.4 POSTPARTUM INFECUNDABILITY

The period between birth and a subsequent conception is constituted by the infecund period and waiting time to conception. Postpartum infecundability is determined by postpartum amenorrhoea due to breastfeeding and postpartum abstinence. Postpartum amenorrhoea, i.e. the period after birth in which no ovulation occurs, is induced by breastfeeding. In the absence of breastfeeding, postpartum amenorrhoea lasts at least one to three months (Leridon, 1993).

Especially the pattern of breastfeeding, i.e. the frequency and duration, is important with regard to the duration of postpartum amenorrhoea. Intense suckling of the baby can postpone the return of menstruation to one to two years (McNeilly, 1993). Some studies indicate five feeds a day as a minimum for

protection against pregnancy (Anderson and Schioler (1982), cited by McNeilly, 1993). More recently, 80 minutes per day, and a minimum of six nursing periods are mentioned to be highly predictive for postpartum amenorrhoea up to 18 months (Stern et al (1986), cited by McNeilly, 1993).

Weaning and complementary feeding of children, thus less frequent and shorter duration of breastfeeding, are associated with shorter durations of postpartum amenorrhoea. In addition, the period of postpartum amenorrhoea might be shorter due to the death of a child when breastfeeding stops (Leridon, 1993).

The role of the nutritional status of women is not well known (Leridon, 1993: 351). Ford and Kim (1993) remark that the prediction of timing of return of fertility after childbirth is not an exact science and suggest that there may be heterogeneity due to other variables such as nutrition. According to Ford and Huffman (1993), the nutritional status of women might affect the duration of postpartum amenorrhoea in two ways. First, malnutrition might affect the reproductive system and thus postpone the return of menstruation. Second, undernourished women might have reduced milk output, which causes their children to suckle more, thus postponing the return of menstruation.

Based on research in Matlab in Bangladesh, Huffman et al. (1978, cited by Meredith, 1993) found a small significant difference in postpartum amenorrhoea for weight-for-height status. Women with highest weight-for-height status had the shortest duration of amenorrhoea. However, the study did not control for duration of breastfeeding. In a later study, Ford and Huffman (1993) found a larger effect of nutritional status of women on amenorrhoea. Women with a higher weight at pregnancy termination had a shorter duration of postpartum amenorrhoea, compared to women with lower weight. Among women weighing more than 44 kg, the mean duration of postpartum amenorrhoea was 13.6 months, among women weighing 38 to 43.9 kg 15.9 months and among those weighting less than 38 kg it was 17.6 months. In India the same relationship was found. The median duration of postpartum amenorrhoea among women weighing less than 40 kg was 13.1 months, among women weighing more than 54 kg 8.2 months (Prema et al. (1981), cited by Ford and Huffman 1993). Meredith (1993) and

Ford and Huffman (1993) conclude that the relationship between nutritional status and fecundability is a complex one. The effect of nutritional status on duration of postpartum amenorrhoea is there, but is small compared to breastfeeding.

Postpartum infecundability is determined not only by postpartum amenorrhoea but also by postpartum abstinence. Abstinence is behavioural in character. The duration of abstinence also depends on the presence of the spouses (e.g., it is relevant to women who deliver in their parents' place and not in their husband's place) and cultural rules on abstinence.

The models of Bongaarts and Potter (1983) and Becker (1993) guide our research on child spacing behaviour. The findings in the earlier studies, as described in this section, will help us in the interpretation of our own findings on child spacing behaviour presented in Chapter 5.

2.2 Decision-making within Context

To answer the second research question on women's and men's perceptions and accompanying decision-making regarding child spacing and other reproductive health events and processes in the life course, as situated in the context in which people live, we adopt the so-called process-context approach (Willekens, 1990 and 1992; De Bruijn, 1992, 1993 and 1999; Hutter, 1998).

The process-context approach is a micro-approach, focusing on the *explanation* of demographic and reproductive health behaviour of people. It is a theoretical framework that includes and relates to other theories in the discipline of demography, among others those by McNicoll (1985, 1989, and 1994) and Greenhalgh (1989, 1994 and 1995). Important additions are the works by North (1994) and Denzau and North (1994) from the perspective of new institutional economics and the studies by D'Andrade (1984; 1995) and D'Andrade and Strauss (1992) based on cognitive anthropology.

2.2.1 Motivation of Behaviour

How do people decide to act in a certain way? Choice often is seen as rational choice. However, following other authors (Simon,

1986; McNicoll, 1989; North, 1994), we emphasize the subjectivity of decision-making. People typically decide and act on incomplete information and with subjectively derived models which they derive from the context in which they live. Human behaviour is motivated within this limiting context. Motivations of people can be identified by their goals (D'Andrade, 1995), i.e. people are goal oriented and deploy strategies in an environment of opportunities and constraints (Greenhalgh, 1989: 442).

Many scientists have identified motives for human behaviour. Some of them assume motives to be more or less universal (e.g. Maslow, 1970), while others (Rokeach, 1973; Lindenberg, 1990; Greenhalgh, 1989; D'Andrade, 1992 and 1995) relate motives additionally to the context in which people live.

Maslow (1970) in identifying the hierarchy of basic needs claims that people's aspiration level is such that once lower order needs (physiological and safety needs) are fulfilled, higher order needs emerge (sense of belonging and love, esteem and self-actualization). He does not claim that these basic needs are universal or ultimate but 'relatively more ultimate, more universal, more basic than the superficial conscious desires' (Maslow, 1970: 54-5). Rokeach (1973) identified end-states or terminal values (for example, happiness, wisdom, equality, freedom, peace and friendship) as having a strong motivational component and guiding human behaviour. Rokeach too believed that all persons, in all places, possess the same values to some degrees, but, additionally he related terminal values to the value system and culture, institutions and personality. Lindenberg (1990: 212), adopting a rational choice theory and identifying two ultimate basic goals (physical well-being and social approval) assumed goals to be aspired by everyone. The means people have to reach these goals, however, are believed to vary according to social position. Greenhalgh (1988), in her study of fertility change in China, identified two basic goals (socio-economic security and mobility). People develop strategies to achieve these goals, thereby, consciously or unconsciously, following norms of the society. The author does not claim that the basic goals are universal, but contends that they are determined 'partly by the political, economic and social institutions . . . and partly by culture' (Greenhalgh, 1988: 637-8).

Similarly, D'Andrade (1995) doubts the universality of human motivation. He states 'every theorist of motivation adds to or subtracts from or redefines the list' and 'there are as many motives as there are relatively autonomous goals'. He assumes some goals to be more universal (such as being healthy, finding security) but allows for situational variability. Within cognitive anthropology the basic idea is that individual behaviour is the outcome of schemas which function as goals and have motivational force and instigate action (D'Andrade, 1992 and 1995).

2.2.2 MOTIVATION AND (CULTURAL) SCHEMAS

What is a schema? A schema is 'a conceptual structure which makes the identification of objects and events possible. Schemas form the reality-defining system of the human and provide information about what states of the world can be and should be pursued'. In other words, 'schemas form the person's internal representation of his/her environment' (D'Andrade, 1992: 33). D'Andrade explains the cognitive paradigm within anthropology as 'what a creature does is, in large part, a function of the creature's internal representation of its environment' (D'Andrade, 1984: 67), i.e. human behaviour is motivated by schemas.

Schemas actually exist for all kind of things: facts, things, events, life stages, and so on (Strauss, 1997: 49). Strauss and D'Andrade (1992), for example, talk about get-in-line-schemas, or get-married-and-have-kids-schemas, go-to-college-and-have-a-career-schemas. Studies in the field of demography, for example, reveal that inherent in schemas on the marriage system in the USA (Quinn 1997) is a shared cultural conception of marriage that has motivational force Chin (1999) identifies schemas on sexuality and gender influencing the risk perception of adolescents on HIV/AIDS and their motivation to protect themselves. Schemas on sexuality, for example, refer to the interpretation of or meaning given to sex as lust, passion or romantic love. Schemas on gender define the meaning of being a woman or a man and related social expectations (social roles). Mason (1992) identified the socio-cultural meaning of children, the meaning of boys being very different from the meaning of

girls. Changing schemas on child rearing and parenthood in USA were described by Harkness et al. (1992) as well. Similarly, while Erikson (1968, cited by De Bruijn, 1999) defined life stages in the life course (childhood, adolescence), these life stages are interpreted and given meaning differently in different societies, for example, India and Bangladesh (Aziz and Maloney, 1985).

Schemas motivate behaviour and prompt action in the following way (D'Andrade, 1992: 30-1 and 1995: 232). Some schemas function as goals. These goal functions of schemas form hierarchies, where interpretation is passed from a lower level to a higher level, and finally the top level where action is determined. This top level consists of 'a person's most general goals', called the master motives or ultimate goals. These can be compared with universal goals as defined by the authors mentioned in the preceding paragraph. D'Andrade discerns, for example, love, security, success, and work. These top-level schemas initiate action autonomously and function as goals. The second level, or middle level of motives consists of schemas for events such as marriage or job. Inherent in these schemas are clusters of powerful goals, which in themselves do not initiate action autonomously. In general, they require other goal-schemas to initiate action. At the lower, third level are schemas for shopping, going to the bank, and so on. These schemas are entirely dependent on higher-level schemas to initiate action.

An example might be useful here. A young Indian woman with a male child visits a health centre (lowest level schema on when or how to come to the centre, whom to consult, how to behave, etc.) because she wants to use a temporary contraceptive method in order to prevent an early subsequent pregnancy. She thinks that the ideal time between two children (second-level schema) is three years. However, another schema on contraceptives (second-level schema) could be that they have many negative side-effects. The ultimate goal or master motive (top-level schema) that might prompt her to actually start using contraceptives could be security, namely she wants to postpone a pregnancy and achieve a birth interval of three years, in order to be able to feed her son and make sure that he will survive, continue the family line, and secure her own status with her family-in-law. Another ultimate goal motivating her not to start using contraceptives could be her

well-being: the use of contraceptives might have negative effects on her health.

Schemas are learned or internalized. They are learned as part of socialization during a person's development (see Holland, 1992). In addition, a very important set of schemas is culturally determined. For example, after delivery, the physical constitution of an Indian woman is described as *hasi may,* literally tender body (Hutter, 1994). *Hasi may* is defined as (= a schema) a period in which women, after the loss of energy and heat during delivery, have to be warmed up. They are considered to be very vulnerable, not only to illnesses but also to, for example, evil spirits. This schema motivates certain behaviour. The postpartum mother is secluded from other people and curtains are drawn around her bed to protect her against infection and spirits; further care is given by family members (often the mother) for example by heating a charcoal fire under the bed and providing heating food such as wheat, sugar and jaggery. The top-level schema or goal motivating the action might be well-being or security.

The example provided not only clarifies what a schema is and how top-level schemas or goals initiate action, but it also indicates that individual cultural schemas (micro level) that motivate behaviour are embedded in the cultural meaning system of a society at large (macro level). Moreover, the importance of the social context, the influence of norms, becomes clear. Human motivation is only realized in social interaction (Strauss, 1992: 1). D'Andrade (1992: 38) emphasizes this by stating, 'It may well be the case that most goals lose their motivational force without the support of significant others.'

Motivation often is thought of as a cognitive process. However, emotions and feelings are also involved (Rokeach, 1973; D'Andrade 1995; Strauss 1992).

2.2.3 ATTITUDES AND BEHAVIOUR

Motivations for behaviour can thus often be identified by their goals, values or end-states, according to Rokeach (1973). He identifies another level comprising attitudes which is located between values (or motivation) and behaviour. Values are seen as the determinants of attitudes and behaviour. According to

Rokeach (1973) values refer to single beliefs and transcend objects and situations, and are thus more general, while attitudes refer to the organization of several beliefs around a specific object or situation.

The relationship between attitude and behaviour, in turn, is worked out in detail in the theory of reasoned action by Ajzen and Fishbein (1980), a value expectancy theory where human beings are assumed to consider the consequences of their behaviour before they actually act. Motivational factors influencing a particular behaviour are captured by the intention to perform that particular behaviour (Ajzen, 1991: 181). The intention to perform a particular behaviour is determined by the relative weight of attitudinal and normative considerations. Attitudes are determined by beliefs about the consequences of that particular behaviour and the evaluation of these consequences. Normative considerations consist of the subjective norm of an individual, i.e. the perceptions of social pressure put on him or her to perform or not to perform the behaviour (Ajzen and Fishbein, 1980: 6). The subjective norm is determined by perceived beliefs of important others and motivation to comply with these others. The theory of Ajzen and Fishbein thus explicitly incorporates the influence of the immediate social context on individual behaviour.

In an extension, the theory of planned behaviour, Ajzen added perceived behavioural control (a concept comparable with perceived self-efficacy as formulated by Bandura, 1982), which consists of 'people's perceptions of the ease or difficulty of performing the behaviour of interest' (Ajzen 1991: 183). A particular behaviour is determined by intention *and* the perceived behavioural control (ability). This means that people's behaviour is strongly influenced by their confidence in their ability to perform it. Intention to behave thus is determined by attitudinal and normative considerations (see above) *and* perceived behavioural control.

Perceived behavioural control is determined by beliefs, i.e. control beliefs. According to Ajzen (1991: 196) these control beliefs may 'partly be based on past experience with the behaviour (thus to be seen in historical time and over the life course). However, they will usually also be influenced by second-

hand information about the behaviour, by the experiences of acquaintances and friends, and by other factors'. Past experiences with the particular behaviour are considered the most important factors affecting perceived behavioural control (see also Bandura, 1986).

In daily life, human behaviour often consists of routine behaviour, i.e. many daily actions (brushing teeth, bath, eating, etc.) are performed without elaborate 'reasoning' or planning. They are just part of daily routine. Life events such as marriage, pregnancy and birth, or migration, however, take place less frequently, sometimes only once in a lifetime. This (rare) kind of behaviour is more likely to result from a process of decision-making (within the context in which people live) in which positive and negative consequences of the action are weighed against each other.

2.2.4 SOCIAL CONTEXT AND CULTURAL MEANING SYSTEM

People typically decide and act on incomplete information which they derive from the context in which they live. This context is a hierarchical multi-level context (Willekens, 1992; De Bruijn, 1993) and includes the ecological and economic contexts (facilitating and inhibiting factors for behaviour), the social context (the immediate environment, institutions) and the cultural context (the cultural meaning system).

The immediate social context in which people live is assumed to play a crucial role as most people 'are more inclined to gather information in their immediate environment rather than elsewhere and will sooner consult sources of information which are easily accessible' (Willekens, 1990: 13-14; Willekens, 1992: 270). The way in which significant others affect individuals' behaviour is captured in the subjective norm described by Ajzen and Fishbein (1980).

The status of an individual and her or his relationships with other people (either in the immediate context or in the macro-context) varies over the life course and is defined within society. The (social) status ascribed to a person, the roles she or he is expected to play, the actions that are considered to be proper, the type of relationships she or he can establish, all are embedded in

the cultural meaning system and reinforced by norms and rules in the society.

At the macro-level, information on which individuals base their decisions and actions is situated in institutions and culture as a meaning-giving system (McNicoll, 1985; Schotter (1986), cited by Willekens, 1992; Willekens, 1992; De Bruijn, 1993; North, 1994).

Institutions can be defined as 'clusters of behavioural rules governing human actions and relationships in recurrent situations' (McNicoll, 1994: 4-5). According to McNicoll (1994), these rules are shared by a group of people, and thus are public, and violations are counteracted with sanctions, either by an external authority or self-imposed. Social pressure and social control motivate people to adapt to the rules (McNicoll, 1994). Institutions are provided with both material and cultural antecedents. That is, institutions are created by people 'to deal with recurrent problems about material realities . . . i.e. institutions emerge from individual-level transactions' (McNicoll, 1994: 6). But institutions are also related to the cultural meaning system in the sense that they are 'manifestations of ideational systems that give some degree of coherence in the cultural domain of symbol and belief' (McNicoll, 1994: 6).

North (1994), similarly embedding individual (economic) decision-making within institutions and belief systems, defines institutions as 'humanly devised constraints that structure human interaction. They are made up of formal constraints (rules, laws, constitutions), informal constraints (norms, conventions, codes of conduct), and their enforcement characteristics' (North, 1994: 366). Rules might be changed in a short period of time, but informal constraints change only gradually.

With respect to reproductive health behaviour, institutions may provide specific information, in the form of health education or Information Education Communication (IEC) activities. This information is thus purposefully supplied to people in order to change their present attitudes and behaviour. In studying how this specific information affects individual (reproductive health) behaviour, the matrix designed by McGuire (1985) is highly relevant. It distinguishes the source of information (who is

delivering the message), the contents of the message (what is told), the channel of communication (e.g., newspapers, television) and the receiver (who receives the education, the target-group).

Culture is here defined as a cultural meaning system through which people adapt to their environment and structure interpersonal activities (D'Andrade, 1984: 116). Four functions of a cultural meaning system can be distinguished:

i. Representational function, i.e. it defines the knowledge and beliefs about the world (what counts as what);
ii. Constructive function, i.e. it creates cultural entities that people adhere to;
iii. Directive function, i.e. it directs behaviour through social pressure and external sanctions and also by intrinsic motivation to conform;
iv. Evocative function, i.e. it evokes certain feelings (D'Andrade, 198: 92-7).

Cultural meaning systems are related to institutions by their directive function and normative properties and sanctions (D'Andrade, 1992: 34). How does the cultural meaning system (at the macro level) relate to the cultural schemas instigating action at the individual (micro level)? A cultural meaning system consists of the cultural schemas that are shared by a group of people. In other words, the cultural schemas at the individual level are embedded in cultural models, which are 'shared cognitive schemas through which human realities are constructed' (Strauss, 1992: 1).

Culture is viewed as a dynamic concept. North (1994) adds the time component within a belief system determining the choices that people make. He defines culture as 'A consequence of learning through time—not just the span of an individual's life or a generation of a society—but the learning embodied in individuals, groups and societies that is cumulative through time and passed inter-generationally by the culture of a society' (North, 1994: 360).

Contextual variables such as economic and ecological circumstances, institutions and cultural meaning systems change and evolve over time, affecting individual decision-making and

individual behaviour. Reproductive behaviour itself evolves over time and generations: younger Indian women, for example, show a different pattern of reproductive behaviour than their mothers.

2.2.5 INTERACTION BETWEEN INDIVIDUAL AND CONTEXT

We thus situate individual behaviour within a multi-hierarchical context. How do the two interact? Evidently, there is interdependency of the individual and the context in which he or she lives. Individual behaviour is determined by the context. The stronger the relationships between a particular meaning system and the institutional context, particularly when they become manifest in formal constraints (laws, rules and constitutions) and are reinforced by social pressure and sanctions, the stronger their influence can be on individual behaviour.

However, individuals are not passive. Although individual behaviour is indeed governed by laws, rules, norms and values, individuals are also active and give shape to institutions and culture (De Bruijn, 1993; McNicoll, 1994; Greenhalgh, 1994). Moreover, individuals do not just follow the regulations, they also try to change the constraints imposed by institutions and the cultural meaning system: they are not just submissive but also try to manipulate information from the context (Strauss, 1992: 13).

The above-mentioned life-course approach and the theories on motivation, cultural schemas, planned behaviour (micro level) as well as those on institutions and cultural meaning systems (macro level) guide our research on decision-making processes regarding child spacing and reproductive health behaviour of women in the context in which they live.

The life course perspective, i.e. situating actual child spacing behaviour within the reproductive health career, is adopted in the whole research. The models developed by Fishbein and Ajzen (1980) and Ajzen (1992) are applied especially in Chapter 7 on attitudes, subjective norm and perceived behavioural control in the use and non-use of modern temporary contraceptives. The concept of cultural schemas and how these schemas lead to and motivate action is applied especially in Chapters 6 to 9.

3

Methodology

Following the research questions, as formulated in the Introduction, and the theoretical framework as worked out in Chapter 2, this chapter describes the research methodology applied. A multi-level research methodology was adopted. A census was conducted in the 11 research villages in Dharwad *taluka* in 1996-7. Based on the census data, women were selected as respondents in a survey conducted in 1997. From the survey, women were selected for participation in in-depth interviews, conducted in 1998. Subsequently, in one of the research villages, in-depth interviews were conducted among male respondents. For details on methodology adopted, see the interim reports of the research project (Hutter, 1998; Rajeswari and Hutter, 1998; Hutter et al., 1999; Hutter et al., 2002).

3.1 Census

In view of our overall main objective to situate child spacing and reproductive health behaviour of Indian women in the changing context in which they live, information on the research area was collected through a household census. The census yielded contextual data especially on the socio-economic status of households and the demographic characteristics of the research population. Because the research was conducted in the same 11 villages of Dharwad *taluka* as an earlier project five years ago (Hutter, 1994), it enabled a comparison in time of the situation in the villages. In the first instance, we wanted to collect data on changes in the household by connecting a particular household in 1991 to its present status. However, this turned out to be an enormous, if not impossible, job. Due to family break-ups,

households were difficult to follow up. To site one example, a joint family consisting of four brothers and their families in 1991 broke up. In 1996-7, each brother had his own nuclear family and lived in a separate house in different neighbourhoods in the village. There were many such instances which made it fairly impossible to follow up the households. At the general level, however, comparisons between the two time periods can be made. For example, the difference in number of households having electricity supply or the number of households owning televisions in both 1991 and 1996-7 can be ascertained.

The basis for the questionnaire employed in the census was the 1991 census. The data on households included common aspects covered in a census such as religion, caste, details of land holding, number of animals owned, type of housing, sources of water supply, type of material used for cooking and household possessions. Also included were details on primary and secondary sources of income. In addition, for all members of the household, data were collected on sex, age, marital status, educational level and occupation. Data on the number of births and deaths during the last one year were collected as well. Information on current family planning status of the members of the household was also obtained.

3.1.1 OPERATIONALIZATION OF VARIABLES

A household was defined as a group of people who prepare their food in the same kitchen and who keep a common household account. Type of household and family was operationalized as in the 1991 census: nuclear or joint and co-residing (more than one household in one house) or single.

The changes that had taken place during the last five years were self-reported. We asked respondents about perceived changes in general economic well-being (improvement, deterioration or same) and perceived causes (economic or family-related). Of course, asking about changes during the last five years is a difficult task. How can people accurately recall events and information pertaining to five years ago? As a reference point the national census in 1991 was taken as well as the assassination

of Rajiv Gandhi in May 1991. In reality, the respondents appeared to recall more easily by associating the year 1991 with the time that a Dutch researcher visited the villages.

Caste was operationalized as caste plus sub-caste. The number of acres owned included acres owned, leased out, cultivated or fallow land, and plantation and excluded acres which were leased in. Encroached land and shared land were discerned separately. Size of land was estimated in acres or *guntas* (40 *guntas* is equal to one acre). Source of income was operationalized as primary and secondary and was, following the earlier census, as specific as possible. That is, for example, not only wage labour was reported but also the kind of wage labour: agricultural, forest department, stone crushing, making leaf-plates, or *gaundi* (construction). Agriculture could be a primary source of income if the household owned the land. Other sources were as detailed as possible, thereby reflecting the Indian context and caste-related jobs, e.g. mat making, bamboo work, fishing, basket making, leather work, begging, *pujari* (priest), and *kaava* (milk product) making by the Goulis tribe.

The total annual income of the household was estimated as follows:

- In the case of a paid job, the salary was considered to be the income per year.
- In the case of agriculture, the number of bags of paddy, quintals of cotton, tons of sugarcane, kilograms or bags of *jola* (sorghum) or pulses was estimated and multiplied by the prices that cultivators got for them, at the time of the present census and five years ago. The information on prices was checked with the Agricultural Producing Marketing Committee (APMC) in Dharwad.
- In the case of wage labour income, daily wages were estimated for males and females, and different types of wage labour. Multiplied by the number of months worked per year and the number of working household members yielded to the annual income of the household. For example, in 1991, women earned Rs. 10 only per day, men Rs. 15. At the time of the present census, these daily wages were Rs. 20 and 25 respectively.

In addition, information was gathered for all members of the household. For under-fives, information on month and year of birth was required. A birth certificate or immunization card (which was not yet issued in 1991) was asked for. If these were not available, which was the case for most under-fives, local calendars were used. An exhaustive list was prepared, for the last six years, with important events such as full and new moon days, festivals, etc. Answers of respondents, e.g. their child was born two days before the festival of Naga Panchami and had just completed 2 years, were checked with this list and the date of birth accordingly recorded.

In addition, for every village a list with important events, e.g. the start of an Anganwadi (kindergarten) school, the first bore-well, the first bus coming to the village, the construction of a temple, was developed so that respondents could relate to the time respective events took place. The age of women was estimated starting from age at menarche (on average the age of 14 years was taken) and subsequently related to marriage and childbirth (see the survey for more details).

Marital status of a household member was operationalized as unmarried, married, separated, deserted, legally divorced, widowed and remarried. In the case of a pre-puberty marriage, the age at consummation of marriages was reported too.

Educational status of each member of the household was operationalized as the highest level of education ever reached and completed. For children, the present standard completed was reported. In addition, those who had not completed primary level education (p_4) were asked whether they could read and write. If they could only write their name and sign, they were not considered to be literate.

Causes of death were self-reported causes.

3.1.2 DATA COLLECTION IN THE FIELD

Members of the team visited all villages to acquaint villagers with the research project. Village leaders, panchayat (village council) members and religious leaders were visited and the aims of the project were explained. Different group leaders, for example, from the Muslims, Jains, Harijans and Bhovis in Mugad, were

visited. The former research, conducted in cooperation with research assistants living in the villages themselves, and the company of some of these research assistants made the first introduction much easier.

Before starting the census, each household in the selected village was numbered. The maps prepared for the earlier study were used as a guideline. On arrival in a new village, one member of the team would number the houses and list the name of head of the household. This separate household enumeration list included particulars on household number, name of the head of the household, official panchayat number (if available) or household number according to the earlier census and interview status for the present study. New maps were prepared with particulars of the names of the different routes/streets and also the location of water-tanks, hand pumps, temples, schools, flour mills, and so on.

The actual data collection took place from 4 October 1996 to 2 January 1997. The data were collected through the personal interview method with the help of a questionnaire. The information was collected either from the head or from the person in-charge of the household. Where the head was not available for interview during the first two visits, data were gathered from the person in-charge.

All the usual residents of the household, i.e. all persons actually living and residing in the household, were enumerated. That means, for example, that married daughters who came to their mother's place for their delivery were not included, but daughters-in-law who had left their husband's place for delivery were included.

3.1.3 COVERAGE

Details on the coverage of households are given in Table 3.1. It must be noted here that although 11 villages are covered, the total number of units in the table amounts to 14. The village of Nagalavi consisted of three different villages or hamlets, at a distance of about 1-2 km from each other. The village Holtikoti had one adjacent hamlet T. Ramachandra Nagar where the resettled Gouli tribe lived (see Chapter 4).

TABLE 3.1: COVERAGE OF HOUSEHOLDS IN THE CENSUS, BY VILLAGE

Village	*Total number of Households*			
	1991 (own) Census		*Current Census*	
	N Covered	*N Listed*	*N Covered*	*% Covered*
Mugad	707	860	839	97.6
Mandihal	193	253	237	93.7
Warava Nagalavi	67	120	117	97.5
Station Nagalavi	26	37	32	86.5
Goutan Nagalavi	20	38	34	89.5
Ramapur	174	271	263	97.0
Veerapur	122	155	152	98.1
Kallapur	123	165	165	100.0
Devar Hubli	300	342	337	98.5
Lalgatti	56	67	62	92.5
Devagiri	67	88	85	96.6
Holtikoti	105	123	113	91.9
T.R. Nagar	22	24	22	91.7
Mavinkoppa	58	71	69	97.2
Total	2,040	2,614	2,527	96.7

The total number of households listed was 2,614 and the coverage was 97 per cent (2,527). As compared to the previous census in 1991, an increase in the number of households ranging between 20 to 35 per cent was applicable to most villages. The growth in population could be attributed to births of children as well as for example, migration of people from Andhra Pradesh to the stone quarries near Mandihal. In addition, the process of families breaking up will have led to the establishment of new households and an increase in the total number of households.

The total coverage in the census is 97 per cent. In one village, Kallapur, the coverage was 100 per cent. Non-coverage was mainly due to non-availability of the head or a responsible person in the household in the day time, seasonal migration and temporary out migration. Only one person refused to participate.

3.2 Survey

The objective of the survey was to collect information regarding actual spacing behaviour and its proximate determinants and to

situate the spacing behaviour within the reproductive health career of women by relating it to other reproductive health events. Pregnancy histories were collected as well as data on first menstruation and marriage. In addition, the survey collected some preliminary information on beliefs and perceptions regarding child spacing and its proximate determinants. More specifically, the survey gathered information on attitudes, subjective norm and perceived behavioural control as delineated developed by Fishbein and Ajzen (1980) and Ajzen (1992) regarding one of the proximate determinants, i.e. contraceptive use. Situating child spacing within the social and cultural context, the survey additionally collects contextual data on the status of women.

Respondents selected for the survey from the census were women who were reported:

(a) to be currently married and in the childbearing age; and
(b) to have at least one surviving child.

Women who were married 15 years or less were selected, thus aiming at a total number of about 1,000 respondents in the survey. The sample of respondents thus consisted of women who had completed their childbearing and were sterilized and women who were still in their childbearing career. Characteristics of the study population are provided in Chapter 4.

3.2.1 OPERATIONALIZATION OF VARIABLES

(a) Estimation of Age and Age at Menarche and Marriage

Age of the respondent is operationalized as either date of birth or the estimated age. As mentioned earlier about the census, it was difficult to get to know the age of the respondents. The age of the respondents as reported in the census was considered to be unreliable, as often the information was not provided by the respondent herself but by the head of the household. Very few women turned out to have birth certificates or to know their dates of birth. The age of most respondents thus had to be estimated.

The estimation of current age of the respondent was done in the following way. Starting from the age at menarche, the duration of time between menarche and the marriage ceremony was estimated, thus providing the age at the marriage ceremony. First menstruation is an event that, in general, is clearly remembered by the women in the survey, as traditionally menarche is the sign that a girl is marriageable. In the local language (Kannada), girls are literally said to become 'big' (*dodakke*). In many religious and caste groups, the event is marked by certain rules and celebrated with a special ceremony (see Chapters 8 and 9). Similarly, marriage is a very important event.

Then, for estimation of the current age of the respondent, the period between the ceremony of marriage and the actual consummation of marriage was estimated. These two events often do not occur at the same time. Also consummation of marriage is an important life event commemorated with special customs (see also Chapter 9), and therefore usually also remembered well.

Subsequently, the period between consummation of marriage and the first pregnancy outcome was estimated. Most women knew exactly how many years and months had passed between these two important life events. Having a first child, thus proving one's fertility, is important. After estimating the periods between the subsequent children, ultimately the age of the respondents was estimated.

In general, the estimated age of all respondents might be a bit on the low side. The method described above depends completely on the estimation of age at menarche. Many respondents indicated that they had their first menstruation at 12 years, which is the socially accepted age at menarche. It is reasonable to assume, see for example, the information in Chapter 2, that 12 years might be a bit too low in this population. But even while probing for more details, e.g. whether a woman was late or early in reaching maturity compared to her friends or girls in her neighbourhood, women found it difficult to give their exact age at the time of menarche. To make it easier for respondents to remember the timing, we first asked whether the family conducted a special ceremony.

Very few women (usually the younger women) knew the exact date of their formal marriage, i.e. the date of the wedding ceremony. Sometimes, the date was written down somewhere on a paper, sometimes family members remembered. One respondent remembered a photograph of herself and her husband on their wedding day with the date written behind. Another respondent looked at the bottom of the steel kitchen utensils she brought at the time of marriage where the date of her wedding was engraved. In most cases, however, age at marriage had to be estimated using the local calendar and the list of important events in the villages (see Section 3.2). The month of the wedding was not so difficult to estimate: most marriages in the research area take place in the wedding season between February and May.

Consummation of marriage, also called effective marriage (*gauna* or *osage* in Kannada), is an even more important event than the wedding itself. It is the first sexual intercourse between husband and wife which has to take place on an auspicious day as determined by an astrologer (see Chapter 9).

Furthermore, we asked whether the marriage was arranged and whether there was a consanguineous relationship between husband and wife. The assumption was that within a consanguineous marriage, inter-spousal communication in reproductive health issues might be easier. Categories of consanguineous relationships were a woman marrying her maternal uncle (*sooder maava*), her maternal cross-cousin (*sooder maavana maga*), her paternal cross-cousin (*sooder atteya maga*), or her parallel cousin (among Muslims) and other more distant relationships.

A question on age of the husband, indicating the age difference between spouses, evoked some hilarious reactions. Respondents often did not know or had to ask family members.

(b) Child Spacing and Proximate Determinants

Child spacing behaviour refers to the duration of birth intervals and the constituting proximate determinants (see Chapter 2). In the local language, the concept of child spacing is indicated by the word *antara*, literally meaning the time gap between the beginning of one event and the end of another event.

A birth interval is defined as the duration in months between two live births. The first birth interval is the interval between consummation of marriage and the first live birth.

The respondents were asked starting from their first pregnancy to enumerate all their pregnancies and the outcomes of these pregnancies. After every pregnancy outcome, the interviewer had to probe and make sure that no pregnancy was forgotten, e.g. a spontaneous abortion between two live births. A pregnancy outcome consists either of a live birth, spontaneous abortion (before 28 weeks of gestation or seven lunar months), still birth (child born dead after 28 weeks of gestation or 7 lunar months) or an induced abortion. Local concepts for the different pregnancy outcomes were employed: a spontaneous abortion as *hotte hoitu* or *hotte mugitu* or *hotte bittu* 'the stomach has gone, finished, died', an induced abortion as *hotte tolesuvudu* 'the stomach has been washed'. All these terms are related to the concept of pregnancy: a pregnant woman is called *avulu hotte li adaale*, literally meaning 'she is with a stomach' (*hotte*). Similarly, a tubectomy is described as *hotte kooyudu* 'the stomach has been cut'. The duration of the pregnancy was reported either in calendar months, but more frequently, as reported by women themselves, in lunar months. A pregnancy of 40 weeks, for example, lasts 10 lunar months.

Postpartum amenorrhoea is defined as the duration, in months, of the period after any pregnancy outcome in which no menstruation takes place. In Kannada, the concept is translated as *mutt-illa*, i.e. 'not having periods'. Postpartum abstinence is operationalized as the period, in months, after any pregnancy outcome, in which husband and wife do not have sexual relationships. First, however, the duration of the stay of the woman in her parents' home (*tavaru mane*) after the delivery of the child was determined. Women in the research area deliver at their parents' home, especially the first delivery, but deliveries of higher parity children also take place there. They return to their husband's house within three or five months after delivery. The completed number of months of the stay in her mother's place was noted. Only then the duration of the period of postpartum abstinence was asked for as the period could coincide with the period of a stay in her mother's place.

Asking questions about postpartum abstinence is a delicate matter. It turned out to be relatively easier because in Kannada one specific concept, i.e. *hasege pathya* 'abstinence from the bed' connotes sexual abstinence. The concept is used for sexual abstinence after delivery, but also for abstinence during religious festivals or illnesses. The concept is very much a part of daily life: doctors, for example, frequently advise patients to observe *hasege pathya*. Still, it was not an easy question to pose. The interviewers were instructed to ask the question only when the respondent was alone, and to make sure that the respondent would not feel embarrassed in front of others and feel ashamed to answer. The interviewers developed certain ways to know, or better to feel, the right moment to ask this particular question, i.e. after some rapport was created with the respondent. Also, it was clearly explained again (as in the beginning of the interview) that the information was collected only for research purposes.

Spousal separation was defined as continuous separation between husband and wife for more than one month, due to work, migration or marital problems.

The use of contraceptives is operationalized as the use of any contraceptive method: tubectomy, laparoscopy, oral pill, IUD, condom, withdrawal, periodic abstinence, herbal methods or others. Again local concepts were used. Both tubectomy and laparoscopy are called operations, not sterilization. Tubectomy is called *hotte kooyudu* 'the stomach has been cut' or *hoolige operation* 'a stitching operation'. Laparoscopy is called *current operation*, the word current referring to the electricity thought to be needed for this operation. The oral pill is commonly described as tablets (*gulge*) or by the brand name Mala-D; IUD is known as Copper-T and *wanki* (a traditional arm-bracelet) or *wanki-panki* or *ungra* (ring) or *baale* (bangle). Condoms are often described by the brand name Nirodh or called *rubber* or *plastic chilla* (bag) or *phucca*. Periodic abstinence had to be described by the interviewers. In the first instance, withdrawal was included as a contraceptive method, but the description of this method became so difficult and created problems with respondents, that it was left out. Herbal methods (*gauti*) were included.

For tubectomy and laparoscopy the date of operation was asked for. By relating it to the last delivery, the data were quite

easy to get: most sterilizations are conducted immediately after delivery and women knew exactly how many days, weeks, or months they waited until they had the sterilization. For temporary methods, the duration of use was asked, the reasons for discontinuation, and possible switch to another method.

(c) Perceptions and Beliefs Regarding Fertility and Child Spacing

Child spacing behaviour is influenced by underlying perceptions and beliefs regarding fertility and child spacing. In the survey, these perceptions were operationalized as the ideal number of children and ideal number of sons and daughters. To study the influence of people in their immediate environment, we also asked 'what, as you believe, do these people (mother-in-law, husband, mother) view as the ideal number of children for you?' Other questions on perceptions related to the ideal length of time between the first and other births and how this ideal birth interval could be achieved.

Perceptions and beliefs regarding the proximate determinants were solicited as well. As we wanted to know whether women themselves are aware of the relationship between postpartum amenorrhoea and breastfeeding, we asked why, according to them, they did not have their periods after delivery. In addition, the women were asked their perception of the ideal duration of postpartum amenorrhoea, breastfeeding and abstinence.

In order to know more about sexual abstinence in general, respondents were asked whether they knew about special days and festivals on which one has to observe *hasege pathya* 'abstinence from the bed'.

Regarding contraceptive use, we asked the women's knowledge of all methods, where these can be obtained and what they cost. Following the model developed by Ajzen and Fishbein (1980) and Ajzen (1991) (see Chapter 2) contraceptive behaviour was operationalized as ever use of any contraceptive method. Intention to use was measured by the question whether the respondent ever considered using a particular method. Attitudes were operationalized as attitudinal beliefs, i.e. the expected consequences of using a particular method. Attitudes were

measured by asking whether respondents found a particular method acceptable for use and concomitant advantages and disadvantages. Moreover, perceived effectiveness (prevention of pregnancy) and convenience of use were included. Particular cultural beliefs such as the oral pill as something which heats up the body, were included as well.

The subjective norm was operationalized as normative beliefs, i.e. the beliefs of important others, in the eyes of the respondents, about their using a particular method. If respondents heard about a particular method, it was asked whether they ever discussed it with someone and with whom. And what, in the respondent's view, would people such as husband, mother-in-law, mother and neighbours think about them using that particular method?

Perceived behavioural control refers to the respondents' perception of the ease or difficulty of using a particular method. Perceived behavioural control was operationalized by two questions: how easy it is to visit the place where contraceptive methods can be obtained, and how easy is it to pay the costs? These turned out to be quite abstract questions for the respondents. What was meant with 'easy to obtain?' They could easily take the bus to the city and visit a health centre, but they had to ask permission from their husbands. The abstract question often was translated into a practical example. This has definitely influenced the answers. The question on costs was much easier to answer.

For these topics, i.e. the attitudinal beliefs, normative beliefs and perceived behavioural control, a three-point scale was used. The interviewer asked the question and then ticked the answer.

(d) Status and Decision-making Power of Women

Child spacing behaviour is viewed within the context in which people live. The census collected information on the socio-economic status of households and the demographic characteristics of the research population. The survey additionally obtained contextual data on decision-making power and status of women, important determinants of reproductive health behaviour. The status of women was determined by their position in the life course. Young Indian women typically live in a

joint family (Hutter, 1994; Malhotra et al., 1995; Oppenheim Mason, 1995a, b) and are dependent on husband and family members in their decision making (Koenig and Foo, 1992; Hutter, 1994). After reviewing Indian literature (Basu, 1989; Koenig and Foo, 1992; Malhotra et al., 1995; Oppenheim Mason 1995a, b; Dharmalingam and Morgan, 1996; Sujatha and Murthy, 1993) and former surveys, the status of women and their decision-making power was operationalized as follows:

- educational level (highest completed level of education);
- occupation of the respondent, income and whether she could keep her own salary and decide what to do with it;
- exposure to information by participation in women's groups or membership of a political party; presence of a radio/television in the house, and whether women themselves were allowed to turn it on.
- freedom to move, within the own village, to the next village or mother's place (*tavaru mane*), and to the market or cinema; whether the respondent had to ask permission and from whom;
- decision-making power regarding buying food items in the market, household expenditures, expenditures for festivals, health visits, education and clothes for children.

3.2.2 DATA COLLECTION IN THE FIELD

Survey data were collected by female interviewers, most of whom were married. During the fieldwork, the respondent was first asked whether the time of the interview was suitable, otherwise the interviewer would come back later or on another day. Sometimes interviews were conducted in the kitchen, the interviewer asking the questions and writing the answers, the respondent making *roti* and vegetable curries. Interviewers addressed the respondents in appropriate local ways. For example, addressing an older woman as *akkara* (*elder sister*) and younger respondents as *tangi* (younger sister).

The interviewers chose a place in the house where both interviewer and respondent could sit and talk, undisturbed by

others. Sometimes, when men were around and it was difficult to ask certain questions, it turned out to be amazingly easy to make the men leave by stating 'it is all about women's business'.

3.2.3 COVERAGE

Table 3.2 provides the details of the survey coverage. According to the census, there were 1,222 currently married women who were married for 15 years or less and had at least one surviving child. In the survey only 951 of these 1,222 women could be interviewed. Thus, the overall coverage was 78 per cent.

Most women who could not be interviewed were not available. They had gone to their native place for a festival or delivery, or migrated temporarily. Four per cent of the women who were identified in the census for participation refused to be included in the survey.

TABLE 3.2: ELIGIBLE WOMEN IDENTIFIED IN THE CENSUS AND THE NUMBER OF WOMEN INTERVIEWED IN THE SURVEY (BY VILLAGE)

	Number of Eligible Women		
Village	*Identified in Census*	*Interviewed*	*Coverage Rate in Survey %*
Mugad	364	298	81.9
Mandihal	111	81	72.9
W. Nagalavi	54	40	74.1
S. Nagalavi	12	8	66.6
G. Nagalavi	22	15	68.2
Ramapur	140	99	70.7
Veerapur	79	59	74.7
Kallapur	91	79	86.8
Devarhubli	154	123	79.9
Lalgatti	39	30	76.9
Devageri	39	31	79.5
Holtikoti	59	48	81.3
T.R.Nagar	17	12	70.6
Mavinkoppa	41	28	68.3
Total	1,222	951	77.8

3.3 In-depth Interviews: Female Perspective

In the second part of the research, we wanted to know about the decision-making processes regarding child spacing and reproductive health behaviour. We wanted to know the perceptions and beliefs (more in-depth than what was covered in the survey), motivation of behaviour and the cultural schemas underlying the behaviour. Therefore, in-depth interviews were conducted.

A list of questions guided the in-depth interviews, starting with menarche, continuing with marriage, and then from first birth interval to first pregnancy and delivery, and ending with sterilization. Reproductive health processes such as menstruation, sexuality, gynaecological morbidity, knowledge about the reproductive system were asked about. An earlier research (Hutter, 1994) already collected information on perceptions about pregnancy and delivery, so these events were excluded.

Perceptions on events in the reproductive health career are additionally related to perceptions of women about their own body and the reproductive system. Ceremonies marking the transitions from one stage in the reproductive health career to another were inquired about, as well as changes (in behaviour, dress, social roles, social expectations) that occur following the particular event, and status and decision-making power of women. Health problems in each of the stages of the reproductive health career and how to deal with them were identified. In addition, we asked about the feelings and emotions of women when they progressed from one stage in the life course to another.

The in-depth interviews thus present the voices of women themselves on reproductive health. The interviews were conducted among women who were selected from the survey. The target groups selected through which the decision-making processes on child spacing could be studied were:

- women who ever used spacing methods; and
- women who never used spacing methods.

Ever use of spacing methods included the use of modern methods such as Copper-T and oral pill (used for at least 12 months), condom, but also so-called abortion tablets, herbal

methods, and periodic abstinence. In this way, we arrived at a total of 33 possible respondents. The sample included women living in different villages, of different religious and caste background, age, educational level, occupation and type of household.

The group of women who had ever used methods were subsequently 'matched' with women who never used these methods. Matching was done with background characteristics of age, educational level, parity, and duration of marriage. In addition, care was taken to ensure that women were selected from different villages, different religious and caste backgrounds, age groups and levels of education.

In order to know how women and couples were influenced in their child spacing and reproductive health decisions by people in their immediate social environment or by health services personnel, a separate list (but almost similar to the one described in the preceding para) guided interviews among key informants. Additional information was also gathered from among mothers and mothers-in-law. We compared their own marital and reproductive health career with that of their daughters or daughters-in-law at present.

3.3.1 DATA COLLECTION IN THE FIELD

The fieldwork was conducted in 1998. All interviews were recorded on tape. In principle, we tried to interview each respondent while she was alone. In the Indian context, however, this is not always possible. Co-sisters or mothers-in-law are usually present in the house. Even if they were not present at the place of the interview itself, remarks from the kitchen or the verandah of others listening could be heard. In most interviews, however, we managed to talk to respondents alone during the major part of the interviews. Starting with general information about pregnancies and children, after 10-15 minutes the by-standers usually disappeared, after which more sensitive topics could be discussed. An interview lasted about 1 to 1.5 hours.

As explained earlier, respondents were asked about their feelings and emotions. Asking directly about feelings and emotions turned out to be more difficult than expected. A very

typical answer to the question 'What did you feel' was 'What is there to feel?' A better way of inquiring about emotions and feelings was through asking the question 'How was it?' Feelings and emotions also could be better identified in an indirect way: the transcripts of the interviews indicate many emotions and feelings expressed by respondents while answering questions on other topics.

The questions about sexuality were not posed to all women. In the first interview it became clear how difficult it is to talk about sexuality and how much rapport had to be established with the respondent before being able to ask questions on an intimate and private topic. A few women were willing to talk about sexuality. It was emphasized again that all information collected was confidential and anonymous.

Comparing the data collected in the census, survey and in-depth interviews, we can observe some clear differences between the different methods. For example, the survey (951 women) indicates more women using spacing methods than the census (2,500 households). Information in the census was collected through the head of the household and in the survey through women themselves. Or, in-depth interviews (37) yielded more information on spontaneous abortions which were not reported in the survey. However, also the reversed happened: the survey reported a few cases of induced abortions about which women did not want to discuss during the in-depth interviews.

3.3.2 COVERAGE

Although we adopted the principle of matching, in reality matching was not so easy: selected women were sometimes not available, had given birth to another child (thus changing parity), so we did not completely succeed in the matching. The group of interviewed women amounted to 37. Of these women, 19 women had ever used spacing methods, and 14 women never used them. Four women were selected as they experienced, according to the survey, special events such as an induced abortion or apparent sub-fecundity.

The interviewed women were of different religions (Hindu,

Muslim, Gouli tribe) and caste backgrounds (Maratha, Lingayat, Brahmin, Jain, Panchal, Kurbar, Valmiki, Uppar, Harijan). Their age ranged from 16 to 31 years. Their educational level was low, only 2 respondents had an educational level as high as SSLC (10th standard). The first group of women, i.e. those who had ever used spacing methods, included relatively more women living in the villages of Mugad and Devarhubli. This is quite logical as the percentage of respondents who ever used spacing methods was higher in these two villages which were located closer to the city of Dharwad.

Key informants interviewed were:

- 8 mothers/mothers-in-law, living in different villages.

Among health providers:

- 3 traditional birth attendants (TBAs),
- 2 Anganwadi workers
- 3 Auxillary-Nurse-Midwives (ANMs)
- 2 traditional healers, one of them an Ayurvedic doctor.

One elderly female Panchayat member and one elderly farmer were interviewed about festivals on fertility and their relationship with the agricultural cycle. In the course of the fieldwork, astrology turned out to play an important role in determining the timing and decisions regarding reproductive health events. Therefore, an astrologer was interviewed as well.

3.3.3 OBSERVATION

In addition to the interviews, observational techniques were applied. Relevant ceremonies and festivals were attended and observations made:

- Rituals to indicate the end of the period of *hasi may* after delivery.
- *Hoolie* festival (burning of Kama) in T. Ramachandra Nagar among the Gouli tribe.
- Several marriage ceremonies:
  - Wedding ceremony in one of the villages.

  - *Ashada karya*: part of the wedding ceremonies.
  - *Hannu idudu* (giving the fruit, i.e. the family of the future bridegroom comes to see the future bride and the marriage is fixed).
  - *Neer madoodu* ceremony: part of wedding ceremony.
  - *Neer madoodu* for child marriage.
  - Preparation for a wedding of three family members (two sons, one daughter of 8 years old).
- Consultation of the *panchanga* and an astrologer, and by a mother whose daughter reached maturity.

3.3.4 Analysis of the Interviews

All the interviews were translated from Kannada into English, while particular concepts and words remained in Kannada. Full transcripts were made. Analysis of the scripts of the interviews was done based on the principles of grounded theory.

3.4 In-depth Interviews: Male Perspective

The main objective of the small study on the male perspective was to understand the perceptions of men and cultural meanings related to various issues surrounding reproductive health in general and sexuality, the reproductive system, gender relationships, and male responsibilities in reproduction, in particular.

For the study among men the village of Holtikoti was selected. The village consists of 123 households, i.e. 596 people who are mostly Hindu. Thirty husbands of the women covered in the survey were interviewed. The interviews were conducted by male researchers.

To build rapport with the village, the interviewers first visited the village head, and talked to him about the nature of the study. Since the villagers knew about the study team, it was easy to relate the objectives of the research with that of the overall objectives of the reproductive health project. In addition, two group meetings (one with married men and the other with unmarried young men) were organized to understand the level of sensitivity associated with questions on sex and sexuality, and

also to explain to the group the rationale for studying the topic among rural men. However, it should be mentioned here that the individual interviews are more suited than group interviews in view of the content of the study.

Typically the interview lasted for an hour. The setting of the interview varied according to the situation in which the respondent felt most comfortable to give the interview. Often the interview was conducted in the evening, after sunset, and as it was summer time, the researchers were asked to conduct the interview outside the house, generally in the backyard, in the open space. The interviewers as well as the respondent would sit out in the backyard on a mat throughout the interview, with no or very little interference from other members of the household or the neighbours.

The first half of the interview generally dealt with subjects that are familiar and close to rural men, including family background, number of persons staying in the house, parents and siblings. Gradually, the subject matter of the interview would move to marriage, how the marriage was fixed, who fixed the marriage, etc. In order to understand the content and mechanism through which the rural men came to know about sex and marriage, questions were asked about premarital discussions of the matter with friends; ideas men had of marriage, women, sex, and family; and premarital sexual experiences.

To understand sexuality within the marriage, the respondent was encouraged to talk about the frequency of sexual intercourse and notions about the same; his understanding of menstruation and pregnancy; practices of sexual abstinence and ideas about postpartum amenorrhoea. The respondents were also probed about the desired number and sex composition of children, about their preference for sons, and about the ideal interval between two births, and how this interval is/can be achieved. The knowledge regarding each method of family planning, his description of the method and his understanding of how these methods prevent pregnancy were also probed.

The interviews, recorded on tape recorder, were translated from Kannada into English by one of the principal investigators. While translating, the Kannada key-words used by the re-

spondents to denote certain reproductive health concepts were retained in the original. Analysis was done based on the principle of grounded theory.

The findings of the male interviews are included in the results of the interviews among women, and are indicated as such.

4

Research Area and Survey Population

This chapter provides background information on the research population living in the 11 research villages (Sections 4.1-4.3) as well as on the survey population (Section 4.5). The first three sections discuss the demographic, socio-economic and socio-cultural aspects of the research area. Data are mainly derived from the household census conducted in 1996-7. Findings indicate that circumstances in the research area have changed. A summary of these changes is provided in Section 4.4. During the intervening five years, India underwent major changes especially in the field of communications and media. This changing environment forms the context against which the survey population is juxtaposed (Section 4.5).

4.1 Demographic Profile of the Research Area

In this section, we describe the demographic characteristics of the research area in the 11 villages, which include the total population and number of households (Section 4.1.1); the age and sex distribution, and marital status (Section 4.1.2); educational background (Section 4.1.3); and fertility, mortality and family planning figures (Section 4.1.4).

4.1.1 Total Population and Households

The research population is distributed over 11 villages (see Table 4.1) or 14 units (Nagalavi consists of one village and two smaller hamlets; Holtikoti has a hamlet T. Ramachandra Nagar where the Gouli tribe lives). In 1991-2, 11,621 inhabitants were enumerated. The population increased to 13,191 in

TABLE 4.1 : RESEARCH AREA: TOTAL POPULATION, NUMBER OF HOUSEHOLDS, AVERAGE SIZE OF THE HOUSEHOLD (BY VILLAGE)

Village	*Total Population*		*Total Households*		*Average Size of the Household*	
	N	%	N	%	*1996-7*	*1991-2*
Mugad	4,336	32.9	839	33.2	5.2	5.5
Mandihal	1,164	8.8	237	9.4	4.9	5.4
W. Nagalavi	545	4.1	117	4.6	4.7	5.3
S. Nagalavi	137	1.0	32	1.3	4.3	5.2
G. Nagalavi	169	1.3	34	1.3	5.0	5.5
Ramapur	1,407	10.7	263	10.4	5.3	6.4
Veerapur	785	6.0	152	6.0	5.2	5.7
Kallapur	870	6.6	165	6.5	5.3	6.2
Devar Hubli	1,777	13.5	337	13.3	5.3	5.5
Lalgatti	331	2.5	62	2.5	5.4	5.5
Devagiri	512	3.9	85	3.4	6.0	6.9
Holtikoti	598	4.5	113	4.5	5.3	5.5
T.R. Nagar	149	1.1	22	0.9	6.9	6.3
Mavinkoppa	411	3.1	69	2.7	6.0	5.9
Total	13,191	100.0	2,527	100.0	5.2	5.7

1996-7, a growth rate of more than 13 per cent.

The research population consists of 2,527 households. The average number of persons living in a household has declined over the five years: from 5.7 in 1991-2 to 5.2 in 1997-8. One reason for this could be the breaking up of joint families into nuclear families (see later).

4.1.2 AGE, SEX AND MARITAL STATUS

The research population is relatively young. The young dependent population, i.e. younger than 15 years, makes up 38 per cent of the total population. Those of working age 15-59 years account for 56 per cent, while about 6 per cent of the total population is aged 60 and above.

The sex ratio of the total population is 943 (see Table 4.2), which is close to the sex ratio for Dharwad rural (948) and

TABLE 4.2: SEX RATIO BY AGE

Age group (years)	*Population N*		*Sex ratio*
	Male	*Female*	
0-4	858	802	935
5-9	878	885	1,008
10-14	835	696	834
15-19	698	620	888
20-4	637	633	994
25-9	565	540	956
30-4	482	487	1,010
35-9	442	378	855
40-4	351	313	892
45-9	279	249	892
50-4	204	217	1,064
55-9	165	177	1,073
60-4	143	159	1,112
65-9	103	113	1,097
70+	147	124	844
NR	3	8	–
Total	6,790	6,401	943

Dharwad district (944) (GOI Census, 1991). It is however lower than for rural Karnataka (975). The sex ratio in the same villages was 922 as per the 1991-2 census.

Half of the total research population is single. About 41 per cent are currently married, while a few people are reported to be separated (0.9 per cent) or to be deserted (0.7 per cent). Widowers make up 6 per cent of the population. Analysis of data on marital status by age reveals that 99 per cent of the population under age 15 years are single. Among those aged 18-21 years, 54 per cent are unmarried while 44 per cent are currently married. The majority of those aged above 21 years are married (75 per cent), and only 6 per cent are unmarried.

More women than men tend to be married. At the age of 20, 76 per cent of women are married. For men, the proportion is 7 per cent only. The proportion of single men is much higher (30 per cent) than for women (10 per cent). But women remain separated (2.4 per cent) and deserted (2.0 per cent) for a longer time as compared to men (only 0.6 and 0.3 respectively).

Moreover, the incidence of widowhood is much higher among women than men, 16.3 per cent against 3.1 per cent. Remarriage is much more common for men (4.3 per cent). Twenty women turned out to have remarried.

Taking the legal minimum age at marriage for girls to be 18 years and for boys 21 years, just 19 per cent of women got married at the legal age, as opposed to 64 per cent of men. Marriages of boys and girls below 12 years are considered as child marriages, and about 8 per cent of the total marriages are child marriages. The occurrence is higher among girls (91 per cent) than boys (9 per cent). The average age at marriage is 23.4 years for men and 16.3 years for women. Exclusion of child marriages results in a marginal increase in the mean age at marriage to 23.7 years for men, while for women it is 17.6 years.

4.1.3 EDUCATIONAL BACKGROUND

The effective literacy rate (with denominator total population aged 7 years and older) indicates that 50 per cent of the total population is illiterate (Table 4.3). About 27 per cent are educated up to primary level (fourth standard completed), and another 12 per cent up to secondary level. Those with with high school education (7 per cent) and college education (3 per cent) are few in number.

Illiteracy among women is very high, 63 per cent against 39 per cent for men. The proportion of men with secondary level

TABLE 4.3: EDUCATIONAL STATUS OF POPULATION (7+) BY SEX

Education	*Male*		*Female*		*Total*	
	N	%	N	%	N	%
Illiterate	2,145	38.6	3,288	62.7	5,433	50.3
Primary	1,777	32.0	1,181	22.5	2,958	27.4
Secondary	787	14.2	541	10.3	1,328	12.3
High School	542	9.8	195	3.7	737	6.8
College	302	5.4	40	0.8	342	3.2
NR	-	-	2	0.0	2	0.0
Total	1,553	100.0	5,247	100.0	10,800	100.0

TABLE 4.4: DISTRIBUTION OF POPULATION (7+) BY EDUCATION AND AGE (PERCENTAGES)

Age Group (years)	Illiterate	Primary	Secondary	High School	College	NR	Total
7-14	22.5	57.8	17.2	2.5	–	–	100.0
15-29	49.9	16.0	13.4	13.6	7.1	0.0	100.0
30-9	63.4	18.5	10.3	5.2	2.6	–	100.0
40-9	61.3	22.1	9.9	4.4	2.2	–	100.0
50+	73.6	18.6	5.8	1.5	0.3	0.1	100.0
Total	50.3	27.4	12.3	6.8	3.2	0.0	100.0

education and above is 29 per cent and just 15 per cent for women.

Nowadays, young people are better educated (Table 4.4). For those aged 7-14 years, 23 per cent are illiterate while for those aged 30-39 years it is 63 per cent and 74 per cent for those aged 50 and above. A much larger proportion of children aged 7-14, compared to the other age groups, have primary education (58 per cent). The proportion with secondary education and above is also considerably higher among the younger population aged 15-29 years.

4.1.4 FERTILITY, MORTALITY AND FAMILY PLANNING

The data in the census indicate a Crude Birth Rate (CBR) in the research area of 27.6 per 1000. This is slightly higher than the CBR for rural Karnataka which is 26.7 (SRS, 1993). The CBR in 1991-2 was 36.7 per 1,000. The Crude Death Rate (CDR) is higher at 10.5 per 1,000. As per SRS estimates it was 8.5 for rural Karnataka in 1993. The death rate was reported to be substantially lower at 6.5 in 1991-2.

Examining the age at death, among the total number of deaths, 12 per cent occurred in the infant stage, 6 per cent between 1 and 4 years, and about one-third between 15 and 49 years. The percentage of infant deaths is slightly higher among boys than girls, while child deaths are relatively higher among girls. The number of deaths, however, is very small. Among those who died at ages 15-49, 48 per cent were men and 52 per cent women. The

slightly higher proportion for women may be due to deaths associated with pregnancy-related causes.

Causes of death were reported by the respondents themselves. The data reveal that old age and related problems account for 19 per cent of deaths, heart attack and heart disease for 9 per cent. Nearly 9 per cent of deaths are reported to be due to asthma and bronchitis. Maternal or delivery problems constitute 4 per cent. Another 4 per cent died due to cancer and 2 per cent died due to blood pressure problems. About 6 per cent of the cases died because of problems related to the nervous system such as paralysis and fits. Suicide and homicide were the reported reason for death 7 per cent of the cases. Of these 11 cases 10 were suicides. In summary, apart from old age problems and suicide and homicide, diseases such as asthma/bronchitis, paralysis/fits, and heart attack seem to be important causes of death, as reported by the respondents themselves.

The census data reveal that among currently married couples, where the wife is in the reproductive ages of 15-49 years, 43 per are practising family planning method/s. For comparison, it was 52 per cent in Dharwad district during 1993-4 (Bhat and Patil, 1994). The acceptance rate varies between 31 per cent in the hamlet T. Ramachandra Nagar to 51 per cent in Veerapur.

Tubectomy is the most popular method, while laproscopy is the choice of 20 per cent of the total users. The number of those who opted for laproscopy is relatively higher in some poorer villages. The acceptance rate for spacing methods (both traditional and modern) accounts, according to the census, for just 1 per cent. It is to be noted that the information is collected from the head of the households and it is highly likely that some users of spacing methods have not disclosed this information to the elders in the family and this might be the reason for underestimated figures (see further Chapter 5).

4.2 Socio-economic Profile of the Research Area

In this section, we examine the socio-economic profile of the 11 villages. We subsequently deal with the settlement structure (Section 2.1.1), the facilities available (Section 2.1.2) and the

economic structure (Section 2.1.3). We will look closely at the changes that have taken place during the five years prior to the second census.

4.2.1 INFRASTRUCTURE OF THE VILLAGES

Overall, the census of 1996-7 indicates some changes in the infrastructure of the 11 research villages, details of which have been discussed by Hutter (1994). For example, roads to some of the villages have improved, tar roads have become more common. In a couple of villages, new Janata plot houses have been built; new poultry farms and stone quarries are now found at the outskirts of villages, especially around Mandihal. In Mugad, the village nearest to the city of Dharwad, many more facilities have been established such as a bank, a veterinary hospital, a public library, more mosques and Anganwadis, lending a more suburban character to the area as compared to 1991-2. The first primary school (up to standard four) was built in T. Ramachandra Nagar, while in Mandihal the primary school was updated from standard four to standard six. The only village that did not yet have electricity in 1991-2, the hamlet Goutan Nagalavi, now has this facility.

A major change is that most villages can be more easily reached as buses are more frequent. Small private buses, so-called *tempos*, provide a means of transportation as well, while in 1991-2 only public transport existed. The villages of Ramapur, Veerapur and Kallapur are still relatively isolated.

The majority of the houses in the research area now have roofs made of tiles. The thatched roof and the roof with mud and stone are slowly disappearing. On some houses, red tiles (considered to be of better quality and to reflect a higher socio-economic status) have replaced the black tiles.

4.2.2 FACILITIES AVAILABLE

Bore water is the main source of drinking water in most villages. It is obtained through hand pumps, public taps and private taps. The number of households with a private tap connection has increased over time. People hardly use any drinking water from a

tank or well (1 per cent). In 1991-2, 13 per cent still used this source of water supply.

There is an obvious increase in the use of electricity. Nearly 65 per cent of the households have an electricity connection as compared to 41 per cent five years back. However, the uptake of electricity is not the same in all villages. Most households still lack toilet facilities, either private or public, and the increase is from 4 to 7 per cent only. Especially the villages near Dharwad, i.e. Mugad and Devar Hubli, have relatively more toilets. Most households still use firewood for cooking (92 per cent). About 3 per cent of the households use kerosene and 3 per cent gas (either *gober* or cooking). Compared to five years ago, not much has changed in this regard.

The number of households owning a radio and a television has increased considerably, from 35 to 46 per cent, and from 2 to 7 per cent, respectively. The possession of a telephone is the privilege of a few households in the villages (N = 22) just as it was in the past (N = 7). Most telephones can be found in Mugad (N = 18) and one household each in the villages of Mandihal, Devar Hubli, Devagiri and Holtikoti.

To summarise in 1996-7 the overall situation in the villages has changed, and there seems to be some development. Not all villages, however, have changed to the same extent. Villages close to Dharwad developed at a faster rate, while the hamlets Goutan Nagalavi and T. Ramachandra Nagar profited less.

4.2.3 ECONOMIC STRUCTURE

For most households, the important sources of income (see Table 4.5) are either cultivation of own land (41 per cent) or daily wage labour (31 per cent). Stone crushing and construction constitute the major source of income for 7 per cent, while about 8 per cent are engaged in modern services, and 4 per cent depend on merchandising.

A comparison of data on primary source of income during the five-year period, as reported by the respondents at the time of the census, indicates that there is a small decline in the proportion of households who depend on cultivation (from 47 to 41 per cent). There is a small increase in the proportion engaged in wage

TABLE 4.5: HOUSEHOLDS BY PRIMARY SOURCE OF INCOME (%)

Primary Source of Income	*1996-7*		*1991-2*	
	N	%	N	%
Cultivating own land	1042	41.2	1174	46.5
Poultry/cattle rearing	9	0.4	7	0.3
Wage labour	793	31.4	755	29.9
Carpenter	46	1.8	46	1.8
Blacksmith	7	0.3	8	0.3
Potter	21	0.8	22	0.9
Rope/broomstick/basket making	26	1.0	26	1.0
Priest	5	0.2	4	0.2
Barber	12	0.5	10	0.4
Dhobi (washerman)	–	–	1	0.0
Stone crushing/building industries	164	6.5	138	5.5
Fishing	26	1.0	28	1.1
Leather work	7	0.3	8	0.3
Merchandise	94	3.7	77	3.0
Modern services	206	8.2	175	6.9
Tailoring	15	0.6	11	0.4
Others	47	1.9	32	1.3
Not working	6	0.2	2	0.1
No source of income	–	–	2	0.1
NR	1	0.0	1	0.0
Total	2,527	100.0	2,527	100.0

labour (from 30 to 31 per cent), stone crushing and construction (from 6 to 7 per cent), merchandising (from 3 to 4 per cent) and modern services (from 7 to 8 per cent).

The changes seem to indicate the start of a trend away from cultivation towards more wage labour, especially non-agricultural wage labour. The figures reflect information provided by panchayat members, who indicated that it was becoming more difficult to find labourers to work in the fields. As transportation facilities improved, more people preferred to be engaged in other daily wage employment such as work in the stone quarries, thereby earning a bit more money.

It is interesting to note that the percentages of households engaged in traditional occupations related to caste such as the blacksmiths, carpenters, potters and barbers remained almost at

the same level. The one *dhobi* (washerman) identified five years back, however, was no longer there.

Overall, agricultural cultivation has become relatively less important in most villages. Some differences between the villages exist. In the villages of Kallapur, Devar Hubli, Lalgatti and Devageri, more than 50 per cent of the households get their income primarily from cultivating their own land. In Goutan Nagalavi, a large majority of the households are engaged in stone crushing work and construction. Modern services are relatively more important in Mugad and Mandihal. In T. Ramachandra Nagar, almost all households are dependent on daily wages. In 1991-2, four households reported to be primarily engaged in cattle rearing and preparation of *kaava* (special sweet made from milk). But in 1996-7 households are no longer engaged in this activity as a primary source of income. Inhabitants indicated that cattle rearing had become very difficult as hardly any grazing grounds were left. More people now migrate temporarily to Goa or Kendra to engage in wage labour work, especially in the construction industry.

Regarding the annual household income, one can observe an increase in the amount of rupees earned. While 6 per cent of the households reported an annual household income of Rs. 4,000 or less, about 49 per cent had an annual income of Rs. 15,000 or more. In 1991-2, these percentages were 13 and 34 per cent, respectively. While the daily wages of agricultural labourers were Rs. 12 to 15 for men and Rs. 10 for women in 1991-2, at the time of the census in 1996-7 these wages had increased to Rs. 25 and Rs. 20 respectively.

Land holding in the research area has remained almost at the same level. A total of 63 per cent of households hold land compared to 62 per cent in 1991-2. The land is mostly dry, i.e. not irrigated. The proportion of households with wet land (irrigated) is small (17 per cent), but higher than the 12 per cent in 1991-2. Also, there is a very small increase (from 2 to 4 per cent) in the proportion of households having a plantation, especially a mango plantation.

In addition to primary source of income, annual income and land holding, respondents were asked about their perception of the changes in income and economic well-being. Of all

respondents, 36 per cent did not perceive any change. A slightly lower proportion, i.e. 34 per cent, perceived an improvement over the five years. About 28 per cent reported that there was deterioration in their economic well-being.

4.3 Socio-cultural Profile of the Research Area

This section describes socio-cultural aspects of the research population such as religion and caste (Section 4.3.1) and the types of families or households that people live in (Section 4.3.2).

4.3.1 Religion and Caste

Hindus constitute an overwhelming majority of the research population (90 per cent), while 9 per cent are Muslim. The Christian population is confined to five households, while a few households belong to the tribal community of the Gouli or Lambani.

Lingayats (27 per cent) and Maratha (21 per cent) are the dominant caste groups (Table 4.6). Next in order are Valmiki (8 per cent) and Kurubar (7 per cent). Jains constitute 5 per cent of the total households. The Voddar caste, traditionally related to stone cutting, also account for 5 per cent. About 4 per cent belong to Madiga or Madar, sub-castes of the Harijans. The number of remaining caste groups is small: the Panchal (craftsmen), either Badiger (carpenter), Pattar (goldsmith), Arkasali (goldsmith) or Vishvakarma, constitute 3 per cent of the households. The number of Brahmin households is only 10.

Some interesting findings have emerged while analysing the data on caste and occupation. Traditionally, caste groups are associated with a particular occupation. This association still exists but is certainly less strong than before. Of the 73 Panchal households, 45 per cent are still primarily engaged in their traditional occupation of carpenter or blacksmith. Of the 21 households that belong to the Kumbar caste, 52 per cent (11) are still primarily engaged in making pots and tiles. The majority of the Bovi are engaged in fishing, but compared to 1991-2 the percentage of people engaged in the fish business has declined. Among 138 Voddar households, 54 per cent are involved in

TABLE 4.6: DISTRIBUTION OF HOUSEHOLDS BY CASTE AND RELIGIOUS GROUPS (%)

Caste Group	*N*	%
Lingayat	684	27.1
Maratha	531	21.0
Valmiki	206	8.2
Kurbar	189	7.5
Jain	126	5.0
Voddar	138	5.5
Madiga/Madar	105	4.2
Panchal	73	2.9
Kshatriya	36	1.4
Bovi	44	1.7
Uppar	32	1.3
Hadpad	5	0.2
Brahmin	10	0.4
Ambiga	18	0.7
Bajantri /Korma/Korwar	17	0.7
Medar	16	0.6
Kumbar	21	0.8
Madiwalar	4	0.2
Muslim	231	9.1
Gouli	22	0.9
Other tribes	4	0.2
Christians	5	0.3
Others	8	0.3
Total	2,527	100.0

traditional stone crushing work. Of the 16 Medar hosueholds, 11 (69 per cent) are still engaged in making ropes, broomsticks and baskets. Just 5 per cent of the Madiga and Madar are still involved in leatherwork. About 40 per cent of the Hadpad households are engaged in the barber trade, while only 16 per cent of the Kurbar still weave. The one Madiwalar, traditionally the *dhobi*, who was still engaged in his profession in 1991-2, is no longer there.

4.3.2 TYPE OF HOUSEHOLD AND FAMILY

Following the 1991-2 study, households are classified into two types, single and co-residing. A single household is defined as a

group of people who prepare their food in one kitchen and who keep a common household account, and who live separately in one house. A co-residing household shares a house with other family-related members. Each household occupies its own part of the house, and keeps a separate household account. In the research area, co-residing households constitute 27 per cent of the total households.

Strictly nuclear families (either single or co-residing) comprising husband, wife and their unmarried children account for 51 per cent. Nearly 27 per cent of all households belong to joint families (either single or co-residing).

Comparing the present data with the 1991-2 data, the proportion of co-residing households has slightly increased from 25 to 27 per cent. The share of nuclear families has increased from 41 to 45 per cent for single households. The percentage of single joint families has decreased from 31 to 26 per cent.

4.4 Changes in the Research Area: A Summary

The data collected in the census in 1996-7 seem to indicate the winds of change in the research area:

- although a high percentage of the population, and especially women, is still illiterate, the younger generation has considerably more education than the older generation; more children go to school in comparison with the past;
- a couple of mud roads to villages have been converted to tar roads;
- a couple of villages have their own school, or have upgraded the level of education of their school;
- the villages can be reached by more buses, including private buses; the most remote villages are still relatively isolated;
- all villages now have electricity; overall more households use electricity;
- more households make use of latrines, especially in the villages near Dharwad city; however, the percentages are still very low;
- more households own a radio, television or telephone;
- the average annual income has increased during the past five years; however, the living costs also have increased and

only 34 per cent of the respondents feel that their economic well-being has improved;

- the proportion of households engaged in agricultural cultivation has slightly declined, while more people work as wage labourers, especially in newly established stone quarries and the construction industry. Improvement in transportation enables wage labourers to seek employment offering higher wages, located at reasonable distance;
- slightly more land is irrigated; also *more* (mango) plantations are established;
- the link between occupation and caste group is still there, but has become less strong;
- there are more nuclear families and fewer joint families.

The aspects outlined above illustrate the nature of the changes. Amidst this changing context, we will situate the survey population.

4.5 The Survey Population

The total number of female respondents in the survey is 951. In Section 4.4.1 we described the characteristics of the community and the households in which the survey respondents live: their religion, caste, socio-economic status and the type of family and household. In Section 4.4.2 we described the personal characteristics of the respondents such as their age, educational level and occupational status.

4.5.1 Community and Household Characteristics

Nearly one-third (31 per cent) of the women live in Mugad village, 13 and 10 per cent in Devar Hubli and Ramapur. The remaining villages each account for less than 10 per cent of the total survey population.

The percentage of households holding land in the survey population (64 per cent) resembles that of the study population at large (63 per cent). Almost half of the households (45 per cent) depend for their primary source of income on cultivation of their own land, while another 33 per cent depend on agricultural wage labour. Wage labour in stone crushing and construction industry

account for 1.4 per cent. Almost 9 per cent are primarily engaged in modern services, and almost 4 per cent in merchandising. Only a small proportion is engaged in activities such as carpentry, blacksmith, pottery, or fishing. The average annual income of the households varies highly, between Rs. 1,000 to Rs. 1,40,000. The households of the survey population are thus, in general, economically a bit better off than the overall study population.

Moreover, with regard to other aspects, the survey population seems to be relatively better off: more than 70 per cent of the households use electricity, as compared to 65 per cent in the study population. Almost 9 per cent has a television (against 7 per cent), 48 per cent have a radio (against 46 per cent), and half of the households (N = 11) that have a telephone (N = 22) are included in the survey.

The distribution according to religion and caste group reflects the distribution of the study population: the majority of the respondents are Hindu (89 per cent), 9.6 per cent Muslim, while 2 women are Christians and 11 belong to the Gouli tribe. Lingayat (28 per cent) and Maratha (20 per cent) are the dominant caste groups. Valmiki and Kurbar each constitute 7 per cent, and Jains, Voddar and Harijans respectively make up 5 per cent of the total. The craftsmen, the Panchal, amount to 3 per cent, the Bovi fishermen to 1 per cent. Only four respondents are bamboo workers and flute players, the Bajantri; two respondents belong to Madiwalar, the traditional washermen caste; and 2 others to the barber caste, the Hadpad. The majority of the Muslims belong to Sheikh and Sayyed sub-groups.

There are some particular differences between the survey and the general study population. For example, the average number of members of a household is higher at 6.8 (against 5.2 in the study population). This is quite understandable, as the survey includes relatively younger women who are married for 15 years or less who tend to live in joint families and have young children. Indeed, the survey population includes relatively more joint families (42 per cent against 27 per cent). Within the age group of 15-19 years, half of the respondents live in a single joint family. With increasing age, the percentage of respondents living in a joint family declines. The percentage of respondents living in single nuclear families is thus very low among women aged

15-19 years (19 per cent). The proportion increases to 31 per cent in the age group 20-24 years, and to 39 and 42 per cent respectively for the age groups 25-29 years and above 30 years.

Most joint families are patrilocal, i.e. the woman live with her husband's family; almost 2 per cent (N = 17) are matrilocal, i.e. the husband lives with his wife's family. Polygamous unions constitute 1.4 per cent of all households.

4.5.2 PERSONAL CHARACTERISTICS

The survey population consists of predominantly younger women, given the selection criteria of 15 years of marriage or less. The youngest respondents (N = 7) are 15 years old, the eldest is 42 years old. Fifteen per cent of the respondents are under the age of 20 years, 37 per cent are between 20 and 24 years, 35 per cent between 25 and 29 years, and 13 per cent of the respondents are aged 30 and over (see Table 4.7). The average age difference between husband and wife is 7 to 8 years.

The educational level (in terms of completed education) of the currently married women is very low. A large majority of the respondents (68 per cent) do not have any education at all. Almost 9 per cent had less than primary education (standard four) while 6 per cent completed primary level. In addition, 13 per cent reached a level below secondary (standard ten, SSLC), while only 3 per cent completed secondary level. Just 1 per cent had a completed educational level above secondary level.

Women who had no education at all and those who had obtained primary level or below, were asked whether they learnt to read and write. Only 5 per cent of these women turned out to be able to read or write. The percentage of illiterate women thus adds up to almost 80 per cent.

Within the group of literate women, the completed educational levels are low. Only three women completed their bachelor's degree, similar numbers for PUC II and PUC I, while 14 per cent completed their secondary education (SSLC). One can observe differences per village in literacy level: in the poorer hamlets of Goutan Nagalavi and T. Ramachandra Nagar, for example, none of the women included in the survey is literate.

TABLE 4.7: DISTRIBUTION OF THE STUDY POPULATION ACCORDING TO AGE AND EDUCATIONAL STATUS

	%		N	
Age (years)				
15-19	15.4		146	
20-24	36.7		349	
25-29	34.8		331	
30+	13.1		125	
Educational Level of Respondents				
No Education	67.9		646	
Below Primary	8.7		83	
Primary Completed (P4)	6.1		58	
Able to Read + Write	(5.0)			
Below Secondary	13.2		126	
Secondary Completed	2.8		27	
Above Secondary	0.9		9	
NA	0.2		2	
Educational Level of Husbands				
No Education	43.3		412	
Below Primary	13.0		124	
Primary Completed (P4)	12.8		122	
Able to Read + Write	(16.5)			
Below Secondary	17.9		170	
Secondary Completed	6.2		59	
Above Secondary	5.4		51	
NA	1.4		13	
Occupation				
Cultivation (Family Farm)	23.9		227	
Wage Labour	32.2		306	
Agricultural		(25.2)		(240)
Non-agricultural		(1.6)		(15)
Stone crushing		(1.7)		(16)
Combination		(3.7)		(35)
Cultivation (Family Farm) + (Wage Labour)	12.5		119	
Household Work	24.0		228	
Other	6.9		66	
NA	0.5		5	
Total	100.00		951	

On average, the husbands of the respondents are better educated. Of all husbands, 43 per cent had no education at all, while 13 per cent had attended primary school and another 13 per cent completed that level. Also, 18 per cent attended secondary school while 6 per cent completed secondary level education. More than 5 per cent had post-secondary education.

Slightly more than half of the women are engaged outside the home, while one-fourth (24 per cent) are housewives. Of all women, 32 per cent are engaged in wage labour, and 24 per cent cultivate their own land. In addition, 25 per cent are engaged in agricultural wage labour, while a minority are engaged in other wage labour employment (such as leaf plate making, broom making) or stone crushing (1.7 per cent). A mere 3 per cent is engaged in a combination of wage labour, while 13 per cent of all women engage in wage labour additional to the cultivation of own land. Just 7 per cent are engaged in salaried employment, such as services, teaching, tailoring, etc.

The analysis of occupation by age provides interesting information: most of the younger respondents in the age group of 15-19 years are engaged in housework (38 per cent), 28 per cent in the cultivation of their own land. While the percentage of women cultivating their own land does not differ much between the age groups, the percentage of women working as wage labourers, or cultivation of own land combined with wage labour, is higher for older women. The percentage of women engaged in other occupations is also highest for the oldest age group of women aged 30 plus. The data indicate that more older women tend to work outside the house than their younger counterparts.

Literate women, on the other hand, work more often in the household (39 per cent against 20 per cent illiterate women) and in other occupations (17 per cent against 4 per cent). More illiterate women are engaged in wage labour—39 per cent against only 8 per cent for literate women—or cultivation of own land plus wage labour (14 per cent against 7 per cent). A conclusion can be that more illiterate women tend to work outside the house in wage labour. If literate women work, it is more often in higher rated occupations such as tailoring and services.

4.6 The Survey Population: A Summary

In summary, the survey population is relatively young which is quite logical given the selection criteria of less than 15 years of marriage. The survey population is economically slightly better off than the total research population. However, literacy level is extremely low: 80 per cent of all women included in the survey cannot read or write. The distribution of religion and caste is similar to the research population. The majority are Hindu, about 9 per cent are Muslim.

Regarding the type of household and family, respondents differ from the total population. The former group live in households with more people than those in the total study population. More women in the survey live in joint families. This is also easy to understand, given the selection criteria: more young married women live with their husband and family-in-law after marriage than older women.

Given the changing socio-economic environment of the research area and the characteristics of the survey population, Chapter 5 situates child spacing behaviour of the survey population within this context.

5

Child Spacing Behaviour within the Reproductive Career

This chapter situates actual child spacing behaviour within the reproductive career of women, and it starts by describing the timing of preceding events in the reproductive career, i.e. the age at menarche (Section 5.1) and marriage (Section 5.2). Menarche marks the physiological start of the reproductive career, and marriage the socially accepted beginning. In India the two events are closely related to each other. Menarche often is celebrated as a *rite de passage* with a special ceremony. Moreover, traditionally, a Hindu marriage should take place as soon as the girl reaches puberty. Nowadays, although the rules are less strict, in the villages the two events are still related to each other. Therefore the duration (in months) between these two events is also studied (Section 5.2.2).

While estimating the duration between two events in the reproductive career, for example the duration between menarche and consummation of marriage from the raw data (indicated by the years and months in which the events took place) the Century Month Code (CMC) was calculated. The National Family Health Survey (NFHS) is followed, where CMC is estimated as the number of months since the start of the century (*NFHS Codebook*: 5), and is calculated as

$$\text{CMC} = (\text{YY event} \times 12) + \text{MM event}$$

where YY event is the year in which the event took place, and MM event the month.

Pregnancy outcomes, as reported in pregnancy histories (see Chapter 3), are determined by the occurrence of outcomes such as live births, stillbirths, and abortions (Section 5.3.1). The duration of birth intervals, according to different background characteristics, are discussed in Section 5.3.2, followed by the proximate determinants, i.e. temporary contraceptive use,

postpartum amenorrhoea and postpartum abstinence. The last event is sterilization which in India often marks the end of the reproductive career of women.

5.1 Timing of Menarche

Three-fourths of all women reported that a special ceremony (*aarti*) was conducted when they reached menarche, indicating the importance of the event. The ceremony was conducted for women in all age groups. The percentage even seems to be a bit higher in the youngest age group (almost 80 per cent) (see Table 5.1). The ceremony was conducted for illiterate and literate

TABLE 5.1: WOMEN FOR WHOM A CEREMONY WAS CONDUCTED AT TIME OF MENARCHE, SELECTED BACKGROUND CHARACTERISTICS (%)

Ceremony Conducted?	*Yes*	*No*	*NA*	*Total Women*
Age Group (years)				
15-19	79.5	20.5		146
20-4	75.4	24.1	0.6	349
25-9	72.2	27.5	0.3	331
30+	76.8	23.3		125
Literacy				
Illiterate	75.6	24.0	0.4	751
Literate	72.7	27.3		198
Religion				
Hindu	77.7	22.1	0.2	847
Muslim	57.1	42.9		91
Christian	50.0	50.0		2
Gouli tribe	27.3	63.6	9.1	12
Some Major Caste Groups				
Vodda	95.8	4.2		48
Harijan	95.5	4.5		44
Jain	93.8	6.3		48
Panchal	92.0	8.0		25
Lingayat	81.5	18.5		270
Maratha	81.8	18.2		192
Brahmin	80.0	20.0		5
Bhovi	69.2	30.8		13
Kumbar	66.7	33.3		12
Valmiki	55.2	44.8		67
Kurbar	53.8	46.2		65
Total	75.3	24.7		951

women alike: 76 and 73 per cent respectively. It is conducted more often among Hindu women (78 per cent), but also for 57 per cent of Muslim women, one of the two Christian women, and three out of ten Gouli women.

Looking at some of the major caste groups, almost all Jain women (94 per cent), Panchal (traditionally the craftsmen: 92 per cent), Vodda (traditionally the stone-crushers: 96 per cent) and Harijans (96 per cent) had a ceremony at the time of menarche. In the caste groups of Brahmins, Lingayats and Marathas, around 80 per cent of the women underwent a ceremony. The percentages are lower, around 50 to 60 per cent, for Kurbar, Kumbar, Bhovi and Valmiki women.

More than half of the women (54 per cent) reported that they reached menarche at the age of 12 years (see also Table 5.4). This average might be bit biased as 12 years is the socially accepted age to reach maturity. Slightly less than one-fourth of the women mentioned the age of 13 years. Menarche before age 11 and after age 15 is very rare: around 3 per cent respectively. The mean age at menarche for the study population is 12.8 years (median: 12 years).

The mean age at menarche increases slightly with increasing age of the women, from 12.4 years among women in the age group 15-19 years and 13.1 years among women in the age group of 30+. It might reflect a decline in age at menarche. Literate women reported a slightly higher age at menarche, 13.1 against 12.7 years for illiterate women. The data of literate women might be a bit more accurate as educated women remembered better when they had their first menstruation: they related it to the standard (class) they were attending at school at that time.

5.2 Marriage

In this section, characteristics of marriages are described, e.g., most marriages are arranged and the importance of consanguineous marriages (Section 5.2.1); the age at time of the wedding, as related to menarche (Section 5.2.2) and the age at consummation of marriage (Section 5.2.3).

5.2.1 Some Characteristics

Most of the marriages of the women (98.5 per cent) were arranged by their parents and family. Thirteen women had a so-called 'love' marriage. In our survey population, about 40 per cent of the women were in a consanguineous marriage (see Table 5.2).

TABLE 5.2: CONSANGUINEOUS MARRIAGES IN THE POPULATION (%)

Having Consanguineous Relationship?	%		*N*	
Yes	40.3		383	
Mother's brother		13.7		130
Mother's brother's son (cross-cousin)		4.8		46
Father's sister's son (cross-cousin)		11.1		106
Parallel cousin		0.4		4
Other relative		10.1		96
No	59.5		566	
NA	0.2		2	
Total	100.0		951	

Of all women, 14 per cent married their mother's brother (maternal uncle: *sooder maava*), 5 per cent their mother's brother's son (*sooder maavana maga*), and 11 per cent their father's sister's son (*sooder atteya maga*). Just 0.4 per cent married a parallel cousin, a more common practice among Muslims.

Consanguineous marriages are relatively more common among the older age group (44 per cent), literate women (42 per cent), Hindus (41 per cent), and the higher socio-economic class (45 per cent).

5.2.2 Timing of Marriage, Related to Menarche

The event of menarche and marriage are closely interrelated in Indian society. We analyse this relationship in detail by examining the durations between the two events. This duration can be measured in two ways: menarche occurring before marriage

(most common) or the wedding ceremony occurring before menarche (so-called child marriages) (see Table 5.3).

TABLE 5.3: DISTRIBUTION OF WOMEN BY AGE AT MENARCHE AND AGE AT MARRIAGE

Age (years)	*Age at Menarche*	*Age at Marriage*	
		Married before Menarche	*Married after Menarche*
5		2.6	
6		1.6	
7		0.7	
8		1.6	
9		0.7	
10		2.1	
11	3.3	2.0	0.2
12	54.1	1.8	3.5
13	23.2	0.3	11.7
14	13.4	0.6	18.8
15	3.8		17.4
16	2.1	0.1	12.3
17	0.2		7.2
18			6.0
19			3.0
20			2.1
21			0.9
22			0.8
23			0.3
24			0.4
25			0.1
26			0.1
NA			0.8
Total Number	951	136	815
%	100	14	86
Mean (years)	12.8	8.6	15.4
Median (years)	12.0	9.0	15.0

(a) First Marriage, then Menarche

Among all women, 14 per cent got married before they reached menarche. The age at their wedding ceremony varied between

1 and 16 years. The mean age at marriage for these women is 8.6 years, the median 9 years. Observations and in-depth information suggest that marriages before menarche often are concluded at the time of another wedding ceremony in the family, thus reducing total marriage costs (see Chapter 9).

The proportion of women who marry before menarche is considerably lower for the older age group: 5 per cent compared to 16 per cent among the younger age group (see Table 5.4). The

TABLE 5.4: PERCENTAGE OF WOMEN WHO GOT MARRIED BEFORE MENARCHE, ACCORDING TO SELECTED BACKGROUND CHARACTERISTICS

	Got Married before Menarche %	*Total*
Age (years)		
15-19	15.8	146
20-4	16.3	349
25-9	15.1	331
30	4.8	125
Education		
Illiterate	15.6	751
Literate	8.6	198
NA		2
Religion		
Hindu	14.8	847
Muslim	5.5	91
Christian	50.0	2
Gouli	45.5	11
Consanguineous Relationship?		
No	8.3	566
Yes	23.2	383
NA		2
Present Occupation		
Cultivation (own land)	17.2	227
Wage labour	14.7	306
Cultivation + wage labour	16.8	119
Household	11.8	228
Others	6.1	66
Total	14.3	951

figure is higher for illiterate women: 16 per cent against 9 per cent among literate women. Among Hindu women 15 per cent married before menarche. Almost half of the Gouli women married before menarche, one of the two Christian women, and 6 per cent of the Muslim women. The percentage is higher among the lower caste groups of Harijans (21 per cent), Valmiki (21 per cent) and Bhovi (23 per cent). But also among the higher placed Maratha, the proportion is a high 18 per cent. Among higher situated caste groups such as Jain (8 per cent), Lingayat (13 per cent), Panchal (12 per cent) and Brahmin (0 per cent) the percentages are lower. Among women in consanguineous relationship, the proportion who marry before menarche is much higher, i.e. 23 per cent, compared to women in a so-called 'new' relationship (8 per cent).

First Menarche, then Marriage

Of all women who married after they reached menarche (N = 815), the majority (60 per cent) got married between 13 and 16 years. The majority of women thus got married before attaining the legal minimum age at marriage of 18 years. The mean age at marriage of the women who married after menarche is 15.4 (median 15 years). For some of these women, however, marriage was consummated some time after the official wedding ceremony.

The next section focuses on timing of the consummation of marriage.

5.2.3 TIMING OF CONSUMMATION OF MARRIAGE

For estimation of the (final) mean age of consummation of marriage, three different groups are distinguished:

1. women who married before menarche and whose marriage was consummated only after they reached maturity;
2. women who married after menarche and went to their husband's house some time after their wedding ceremony; and
3. women who stayed in their husband's house immediately

TABLE 5.5: MEAN AGE AT MARRIAGE AND CONSUMMATION OF MARRIAGE

	Mean	*Median*	*N*
Women who Married before Menarche			
Age Marriage (years), at wedding ceremony	8.6	9.0	136
Duration (months) menarche – Consummation Marriage	12.5	10.0	
Age at Consummation of Marriage (years)	13.8	13.7	
Women who Married after Menarche (all)			
Age at Marriage (years), wedding ceremony	15.4	15.0	815
Women who Consummated Marriage Some Time after Wedding Ceremony (out of 815)			38
Duration (months) wedding – *Gauna*	5.3	3.0	
Age at Consummation of Marriage (years)	15.1	14.5	
Women who Consummated Marriage Immediately after Wedding Ceremony (out of 815)			777
Age at Consummation of Marriage (years)	15.4	15.0	
All Women			
Age at Consummation of Marriage (years)	15.2	15.0	951

after the conclusion of the wedding ceremony (see Table 5.5).

In general, girls who married before menarche return to their parents' house and leave for their husband's house only after they reached maturity. For women who married before menarche (N = 136), the average duration between the event of menarche and consummation of marriage (estimated by the difference in CMCs for both events) is 12.5 months (median 10 months). Only a few women (6 per cent) went to their husband's place immediately after they reached menarche. Age heaping is observed at 3, 6 and 12 months. For one respondent the period is as long as 72 months, i.e. 6 years. Overall, one year after having

reached menarche, two-thirds of these women have consummated their marriage. Adding the time between menarche and consummation of marriage to the age at menarche for these women, the mean age at consummation of marriage for these women is estimated to be 13.8 years.

As mentioned above, 815 women married after they had reached menarche. Some of them (N = 38) stayed at home after their wedding ceremony before their marriage was actually consummated, the so-called *gauna*. This period varied between 0 and 24 months, the median being 3 months. The CMC data indicate a mean duration of time between the two events of marriage and consummation of marriage of 5.3 months. Quite some women (28 per cent) consummated their marriage within one month. Adding the time duration between the events of the wedding ceremony and consummation of marriage, the mean age at consummation of marriage for these women is 15.1 years.

The average age of women whose marriage was consummated almost immediately after the wedding ceremony (N = 777) is 15.4 years.

Adding all three groups of women, the mean age at consummation of marriage for the total survey population is 15.2 years.

Looking at consummation of marriage and different background factors (see Table 5.6), the mean age at consummation of marriage is lowest for women in the youngest age group (14.3 years), compared to women in the 30+ age group (17.1 years). This of course is due to the outcome of a selection effect.

Literate women consummate their marriage at later ages (16.8 years) compared to illiterate women (14.8 years). Women in a consanguineous marriage are at a slightly lower age when their marriage is consummated (15.0 years), compared to women in a so-called 'new' relationship (15.3 years). Christian women consummate their marriage at the latest ages (19.2 years). However, there were only two of such women. Hindus consummate marriage on average at 15.1 years, Muslims at 15.7 years and Gouli at 15.6 years.

In conclusion, the women in the survey population married at an early age, on average at 15.2 years. The events of menarche

TABLE 5.6: MEAN AGE AT CONSUMMATION OF MARRIAGE BY AGE GROUP, LITERACY RATE, RELIGION AND PRESENT OCCUPATION

	Mean age	N
Age Group (years)		
15-19	14.3	145
20-4	14.9	342
25-9	15.2	325
30+	17.1	124
Literacy		
Illiterate	14.8	739
Literate	16.8	195
Consanguineous Relationship?		
No	15.3	555
Yes	14.9	379
Religion		
Hindu	15.1	835
Muslim	15.7	89
Christian	19.2	2
Gouli tribe	15.6	10
Present Occupation		
Cultivation (Own land)	15.1	222
Wage labour	14.5	302
Cultivation + wage labour	15.1	115
Household	15.8	226
Others	17.0	66
Total	15.2	936

and consummation of marriage were closely related: for women who married before menarche, for example, the average duration between the timing of menarche and consummation of marriage was only 10 months.

5.3 Fertility and Child Spacing Behaviour

In this section we discuss actual fertility and child spacing behaviour: pregnancy outcomes (Section 5.3.1), duration of birth intervals (Section 5.3.2) and the proximate determinants of fertility and birth intervals (Sections 5.3.3–5.3.5).

5.3.1 PREGNANCY OUTCOMES

The 951 women included in the survey had on average about three pregnancies (Table 5.7). The average number of children ever born in the study sample is 2.7 children per woman. However, only 2.5 children, on an average, survive.

TABLE 5.7: MEAN NUMBER OF PREGNANCIES BY SPECIFIC OUTCOMES, ACCORDING TO AGE OF THE WOMEN

	Current Age			
	15-19	*20-9*	*30+*	*Total*
Total Pregnancies	1.61	3.10	3.84	2.97
Foetal Loss				
Stillbirth	0.03	0.08	0.06	0.07
Spontaneous abortion	0.11	0.14	0.23	0.15
Induced abortion	0.01	0.02	0.03	0.02
Children Ever Born	1.46	2.86	3.51	2.73
Child loss	0.07	0.26	0.32	0.24
Children surviving	1.39	2.60	3.19	2.49

Most pregnancies (92 per cent) resulted in live births (Table 5.8). The proportion of pregnancies that ended in spontaneous abortions (5 per cent) is greater than the proportion of stillbirths (2 per cent) or induced abortions (less than 1 per cent). The proportion of pregnancies ending in foetal loss increases with the increase in the maternal age at conception although it does not vary much by order of pregnancy.

The 5 per cent pregnancies that ended in a spontaneous abortion do not seem to be too extreme. Studies reviewed in Chapter 2 indeed indicate a lower percentage of 2.5 (of all life births) (Singh and Wulf, 1994), but others [Roman and Stevenson (1983); Harlap et al. (1980); cited by Den Draak, 2003] indicate higher percentages of spontaneous abortion, i.e. between 10 and more than 20 per cent. The proportion of stillbirths (2.5 per cent) does seem to be a bit high compared to SRS data of 0.9 per cent (of all live births) for all India (1994) and 1.5 per cent for Karnataka [Rayan and Mohanachandran (1999), cited by Den Draak, 2003].

TABLE 5.8: PER CENT DISTRIBUTION OF LIFETIME PREGNANCIES BY OUTCOME, ACCORDING TO SELECTED BACKGROUND CHARACTERISTICS

Background Characteristics	*Live Birth*	*Still Birth*	*Sponta-neous Abortion*	*Induced Abortion*	*Total*	*Number*
Maternal Age at Conception						
15-19	91.4	2.2	5.5	1.0	100.0	510
20-9	93.1	1.9	4.4	0.6	100.0	634
30 +	84.6	0.0	11.5	3.8	100.0	26
Order of Pregnancy						
1	92.2	2.5	5.3	0.0	100.0	952
2	91.8	2.2	5.4	0.6	100.0	789
3	92.3	1.6	5.1	1.1	100.0	571
4 +	92.1	2.8	4.2	1.0	100.0	505
Total	92.1	2.3	5.1	0.6	100.0	2,817

Overall, 74 per cent of the total pregnancy outcomes occurred at home, either at in-laws' home (23 per cent) or parents' home (50 per cent). It is a tradition in most parts of south India to have the delivery of the first one or two pregnancies in the woman's parents' home (*tavaru mane*). In the research area, in reality, women up to parity five go to their parents' house for delivery.

Little over one-fourth of the pregnancy terminations took place in a medical facility. It is interesting to note that a greater proportion of pregnancy terminations took place in a health facility when the woman was at her parents' place (21 per cent), compared to their counterparts who stayed at her in-laws' place (5 per cent). For 71 per cent of all pregnancies, women went to their parents' house for delivery, and about one-third of such deliveries took place in a medical facility. On the other hand, of the 28 per cent of all pregnancies where the woman stayed in her husband's place, only one-sixth were terminated in a health facility. Younger women and women pregnant for the first time are more likely to have their delivery at their parents' home and at a medical facility than older women and women with higher order pregnancies.

Interestingly, the custom of going to the parents' house during pregnancy (i.e. the proportion of pregnancies for which women went to their parents' place for delivery) does not vary much by literacy and level of education.

5.3.2 DURATION OF BIRTH INTERVALS

The present section describes actual child spacing behaviour, i.e. the duration of birth intervals, related to background factors such as age and parity, survival of the previous pregnancy and sex of the child. In addition, the constituting proximate determinants postpartum amenorrhoea, breastfeeding, postpartum abstinence, and use of contraceptives are described.

Table 5.9 presents the distribution of second and higher-order births (live births) in the five years prior to the survey by the interval since previous birth (live birth). Overall, 9 per cent of the births occurred within 18 months, 29 per cent within 24 months. The mean birth interval is 32 months or about 2.6 years.

The relatively short mean birth interval for women aged 15-19 (24.4 months) probably results from a selection effect. Only women who have had two or more births are included, and women aged 15-19 with two or more births are generally likely to be more fecund than their counterparts of similar age. Differences in fecundability by age of the mother may likewise account for the increase in birth interval by current maternal age. Although the age of the woman and the birth order are positively correlated, the birth interval decreases with increase in the birth order. This is because women with a large number of births are probably more fecund and hence have shorter birth intervals.

The mean birth interval is three to four months shorter when the last birth was a stillbirth or when the infant died (28.1 months) than when the last birth survived (32.4 months). Very short birth intervals are unusually high for the former group (49 per cent occurring within 24 months versus 27 per cent). This probably reflects the cessation of breastfeeding when the child dies and the consequent shortening of the period of postpartum amenorrhoea. Similar findings are observed on birth intervals where a pregnancy between births was interrupted either through abortion (spontaneous or induced) or stillbirth. Birth intervals

TABLE 5.9: DISTRIBUTION OF SECOND/HIGHER-ORDER BIRTHS IN THE FIVE YEARS PRIOR TO THE SURVEY BY INTERVAL SINCE PREVIOUS BIRTH, ACCORDING TO SELECTED BACKGROUND CHARACTERISTICS

Background characteristic	*Months since Previous Birth*						*Total*	*Mean*	N
	<12	*12-17*	*18-23*	*24-35*	*36-47*	*48+*			
Current Maternal Age									
15-19	3.0	14.9	29.9	35.8	10.5	6.0	100.0	24.37	67
20-4	0.3	7.7	23.7	38.6	16.5	13.3	100.0	30.44	376
25-9	1.4	5.0	16.1	37.3	20.4	19.7	100.0	34.93	279
30+	2.8	5.6	9.9	39.4	19.7	22.5	100.0	35.63	71
Order of Prior Birth									
1	0.4	11.2	19.4	37.2	19.0	12.8	100.0	32.05	242
2	0.8	6.2	18.7	36.1	18.7	19.5	100.0	33.06	241
3	0.0	2.8	21.0	39.2	19.9	17.1	100.0	33.22	176
4	3.5	4.7	22.1	46.5	9.3	14.0	100.0	29.38	86
5+	6.3	12.5	27.2	31.3	12.5	10.4	100.0	26.17	48
Sex of Prior Birth									
Female	1.0	7.2	19.6	38.5	17.3	16.3	100.0	31.51	387
Male	1.2	7.1	20.9	37.4	18.0	15.3	100.0	32.41	406
Survival of Prior Birth									
Still living	0.7	6.3	19.6	38.8	18.4	16.3	100.0	32.38	719
Deceased	5.4	16.2	27.0	29.7	10.8	10.8	100.0	28.05	74

Contd.

TABLE 5.9 (Contd.)

Background characteristic	*Months since Previous Birth*						*Total*	*Mean*	N
	<12	*12-17*	*18-23*	*24-35*	*36-47*	*48+*			
Prior Pregnancy Interrupted									
Yes	0.0	0.0	0.0	0.0	0.0	100.0	100.0	45.20	50
No	1.2	7.7	21.7	40.5	18.8	10.1	100.0	31.08	743
Maternal Education									
Illiterate	1.2	6.5	20.4	38.7	18.3	15.0	100.0	32.20	574
Primary	0.9	7.6	15.1	38.7	14.2	23.6	100.0	33.10	106
Primary+	0.9	10.6	24.7	33.6	17.7	12.4	100.0	29.70	113
Use of FP Between Births									
Yes	0.0	5.9	8.8	38.2	35.3	11.8	100.0	34.44	34
No	1.2	7.3	20.8	37.9	16.9	15.9	100.0	31.86	759
Amenorrhoea Between Births									
<5 months	1.6	16.1	26.2	32.7	11.7	11.7	100.0	28.20	248
5-9 months	1.1	6.0	30.1	36.1	14.2	12.6	100.0	29.50	183
10-14 months	1.2	1.2	15.4	44.1	20.1	18.1	100.0	34.30	254
15+ months	0.0	2.8	1.9	38.9	31.5	25.0	100.0	39.50	108
Duration of Breastfeeding Between Births									
<10 months	3.4	23.1	26.9	31.7	9.6	4.8	100.0	24.22	104
10-14 months	1.7	13.6	26.7	36.4	11.4	10.2	100.0	27.80	176
15-19 months	0.6	2.7	28.4	45.9	10.9	11.5	100.0	29.70	183
20-4 months	0.0	1.0	13.3	43.4	20.9	21.4	100.0	35.00	196
25+ months	0.8	1.5	6.0	26.1	36.6	29.1	100.0	42.07	134

Sexual Abstinence following Prior Birth									
<5 months	2.3	10.0	24.6	36.0	14.9	12.9	100.0	29.55	350
5-9 months	0.3	5.9	17.3	40.2	18.9	17.5	100.0	33.09	371
10+ months	0.0	0.0	15.3	36.1	25.0	23.6	100.0	38.00	72
Stay in mother's house following the prior birth									
0 month	2.7	6.3	22.3	40.2	15.6	13.0	100.0	30.41	224
1-3 months	0.9	9.3	19.6	42.2	14.7	19.2	100.0	30.64	225
4+ months	0.3	6.4	19.5	33.7	20.9	13.3	100.0	33.86	344
Total	1.9	7.2	20.3	38.0	17.7	15.8	100.0	31.97	793

vary little by the sex of the prior birth (31.5 months after a girl, 32.4 after a boy) and education of the mother.

The use of modern spacing methods is very rare in rural India. In the survey population, out of the total 793 births during the last five years, the parents of only 34 births were using some contraception following their previous birth. Births to parents who used contraception following the previous birth are about 3 months longer in interval (34.4 months) than births to parents who did not use any contraception (31.9 months). The inherent relationship between the duration of breastfeeding, amenorrhoea, and birth interval is evident as the last-mentioned exhibits a steady increase with an increase in duration of amenorrhoea and breastfeeding. Children born to mothers who breastfed their previous child for longer than 20 months are born at a birth interval of 35 months or longer. The interval was shorter (24 months) for mothers who breastfed their previous child for less than 10 months.

The duration of sexual abstinence following childbirth also determines how soon the next child is born. The mean birth interval is about eight months longer (38 months) if the couple abstained for 10 or more months after childbirth than when the couple resumed sexual relations within 5 months of childbirth (29.6 months).

The birth interval does not differ much for mothers who stayed at their parental home for less than 3 months following the previous birth (30.6 months) and for those mothers who did not go to their parental home for the previous delivery (30.4 months). However, birth intervals are longer (33.9 months) for mothers who did not return to their in-laws' home for four or more months.

5.2.3 USE OF SPACING METHODS

Only 22 of the women (2.3 per cent) were currently using a modern spacing method. In addition, 44.4 per cent of the women were sterilized (either tubectomy or laproscopy). The Contraceptive Prevalence Rate (CPR: here only for modern contraceptive methods) is thus 46.7 per cent.

When all the women were asked whether they ever used any contraceptive methods, almost half of them (48 per cent) responded negatively: they had never used any method (see Table 5.10).

The rate of spacing methods ever used is very low: 2.2 per cent (N = 21) used the oral pill, 1.7 per cent Copper-T, and 0.6 per cent condom. A few women reported the use of tablets for induced abortion, one respondent an injection, and four women the application of periodic abstinence. Seven women used other methods, mainly herbal. In total, only 10.2 per cent of all women ever used a spacing method.

Considering the data for all births (N = 2821), the parents of 109 births ever used a spacing method (including periodic abstinence, herbal methods, and others). For all births, the oral pill was reported to be used 51 times (2 per cent), Copper-T 31 times (1 per cent), condoms 10 times, periodic abstinence 6 times,

TABLE 5.10: WOMEN WHO EVER USED ANY CONTRACEPTIVE METHODS (%)

	%	N
Never Used	48.2	458
Ever Used		
Tubectomy only	34.0	323
Laparoscopy only	6.3	60
Oral pill only	2.2	21
Copper-T only	1.7	16
Condom only	0.6	6
Periodic abstinence	0.4	4
Operation + Oral pill	1.2	11
Operation + Copper-T	1.3	12
Operation + Tablets for induced abortion	0.3	3
Operation + Several spacing methods	1.3	12
Injection and tablets for induced abortion	0.1	1
Oral pill, Copper-T and condom	0.3	3
Other	0.8	7
Vasectomy	0.1	1
NA	1.6	15
Total	100.0	951

herbal methods 3 times, and other methods such as tablets for induced abortion and injection 8 times.

In conclusion, the use of modern spacing methods is very low. And data on duration of use suggests that actual use is even lower (see Table 5.11). Of the 51 times that the oral pill was reported to be used, in 14 per cent of the cases the duration of use was less than one month. Several women mentioned they took the oral pill only for two or three days, one respondent even used it only once. In addition, 52 per cent of the cases stopped using the oral pill within 3 months, 70 per cent within 6 months. The longest duration of use of oral pill is 40 months. Overall, the mean duration of use of oral pill is 7.3 months, the median 3 months.

The situation for Copper-T is only slightly different. Of the 31 times that Copper-T was used, in 32 per cent of the cases IUD was removed within 3 months, 71 per cent within one year, 90 per cent within two years. Overall, the mean duration of use of Copper-T is 11.1 months, a median of 6 months.

There are only 10 cases of condom use: the mean duration of use is 4.3 months, the median 3 months. For the 6 cases of periodic abstinence, the duration varied between 3 months and 24 months. The duration of herbal methods use was about 3 months.

TABLE 5.11: CUMULATIVE PERCENTAGE OF USE OF ORAL PILL, COPPER-T AND CONDOM, ACCORDING TO DURATION OF USE (IN MONTHS)

	Oral pill	*Copper-T*	*Condom*
Duration of Use (months)			
0	14.0	12.9	11.1
1	30.0	16.1	33.3
3	53.0	32.2	55.6
6	70.0	51.6	77.8
12	86.0	71.0	100.0
18	88.0	74.2	
24	94.0	90.3	
40	100.0		
48	100.0		
N	51	31	10
Mean Duration (months)	7.28	11.2	4.33
Median (months)	3.00	6.00	3.00

Another important conclusion here is that spacing methods are especially used after the birth of a first child. In the interval between marriage and first child only one respondent reported to have used a spacing method.

All women who ever used any spacing method are grouped together (N = 93) according to selected background characteristics (Table 5.12). The data show that none of the women living in the poorer hamlets of Goutan Nagalavi and T. Ramachandra Nagar ever used any spacing method. The highest proportion of women who ever used spacing methods are in Warava Nagalavi (15 per cent), Lalgatti (13 per cent), Station Nagalavi (13 per cent), Mugad (12 per cent) and Devar Hubli (12 per cent).

TABLE 5.12: SELECTED CHARACTERISTICS OF WOMEN WHO EVER USED SPACING METHODS AND WHO ARE STERILIZED

		Ever Used Spacing	*Being Sterilized*	N
Village				
Mugad		12.4	39.6	298
Mandihal		9.9	49.4	81
Warava Nagalavi		15.0	52.5	40
Station Nagalavi		12.5	25.0	8
Goutan Nagalavi		–	20.0	15
Ramapur		5.1	55.6	99
Veerapur		5.1	57.6	59
Kallapur		7.6	48.1	79
Devar Hubli		12.2	43.9	123
Lalgatti		13.3	36.7	30
Devageri		3.2	25.8	31
Holtikoti		6.3	41.7	48
T.R. Nagar		–	33.3	12
Mavinkoppa		14.3	50.0	28
Religion				
Hindu		9.7	45.5	847
Muslim		12.1	36.3	91
Christian		–	–	2
Gouli		–	36.4	11
Type of Family/Household				
Single	Nuclear	9.5	53.9	317
	Joint	9.2	36.1	327
	Other	10.4	39.6	48

Contd.

TABLE 5.12 (Contd.)

		Ever Used Spacing	Being Sterilized	N
Co-residing	Nuclear	11.5	48.9	174
	Joint	8.0	34.7	75
	Other	20.0	30.0	10
Age Group (years)				
15-19		3.4	6.2	146
20-4		11.2	31.8	349
25-9		10.9	60.7	331
30+		10.4	80.8	125
Literacy Level				
Illiterate		6.4	44.2	751
Literate		22.7	45.5	198
Present Occupation				
Cultivation		6.6	44.1	27
Wage labour		5.6	50.7	306
Cultivation + wage labour		5.9	40.3	119
Household		16.7	36.4	228
Other		22.7	51.5	66
Total		9.8	44.4	951

It is noteworthy that more Muslim women (12 per cent) ever used a spacing method. Neither the Gouli women, nor the Christian women ever used a spacing method. In age groups older than 20 years, spacing methods are used to a similar extent (around 10-11 per cent). More literate women (23 per cent) used spacing methods than illiterate women (6 per cent).

It is clear that the use of spacing methods is very low in the research area and thus does not contribute much to the duration of birth intervals. As already indicated in Section 5.3.1, the proximate determinant induced abortion also does not play a major role. Other proximate determinants of the length of birth interval are postpartum amenorrhoea and postpartum abstinence.

5.3.4 DURATION OF POSTPARTUM AMENORRHOEA

The duration of postpartum amenorrhoea following a birth is closely associated with the duration of breastfeeding, which tends

to suppress the resumption of ovulation. Table 5.13 presents the distribution of second and higher-order births during the five-year period preceding the survey by duration of amenorrhoea

TABLE 5.13: SELECTED CHARACTERISTICS OF WOMEN AND SECOND- AND HIGHER-ORDER BIRTHS DURING THE FIVE YEARS PRIOR TO THE SURVEY, BY REPORTED DURATION OF AMENORRHOEA SINCE PREVIOUS BIRTH (%)

Background Characteristic	*Months Amenorrhoeic*				*Total*	*Mean*	*N*
	<5	*5-9*	*10-14*	*15+*			
Current Maternal Age							
15-19	46.3	34.3	14.9	4.5	100.0	5.76	67
20-4	34.3	24.2	31.1	10.4	100.0	8.00	376
25-9	26.5	18.6	35.5	19.4	100.0	9.95	279
30+	19.7	23.9	39.4	16.9	100.0	10.30	71
Order of Prior Birth							
1	39.7	21.5	28.9	9.9	100.0	7.59	242
2	28.2	25.3	30.7	15.8	100.0	9.01	241
3	22.7	21.6	36.9	18.8	100.0	10.41	176
4	32.6	22.1	34.9	10.5	100.0	8.00	86
5+	33.3	27.1	31.3	8.3	100.0	7.77	48
Sex of Prior Birth							
Female	30.8	22.5	32.0	14.7	100.0	8.93	387
Male	31.8	23.7	32.0	12.6	100.0	8.48	406
Survival of Prior Birth							
Still living	28.9	23.0	33.8	14.3	100.0	9.04	719
Deceased	54.1	24.3	14.9	6.8	100.0	5.39	74
Prior Pregnancy Interrupted							
Yes	36.0	28.0	26.0	10.0	100.0	7.92	50
No	31.0	22.8	32.4	13.9	100.0	8.76	743
Maternal Education							
Illiterate	32.5	21.6	32.4	13.4	100.0	8.57	574
Primary	23.6	23.6	35.9	17.0	100.0	10.42	106
Primary+	31.9	30.1	26.6	11.5	100.0	7.77	113
Use of FP between Births							
Yes	32.4	26.5	32.4	8.8	100.0	8.29	34
No	31.2	22.9	32.0	13.8	100.0	8.72	759

Contd.

TABLE 5.13 (Contd.)

Background Characteristic	*Months Amenorrhoeic*				*Total*	*Mean*	*N*
	<5	*5-9*	*10-14*	*15+*			
Duration of Breastfeeding between Births							
<10 months	52.9	23.1	21.2	2.9	100.0	5.37	104
10-14 months	31.3	27.3	31.8	9.7	100.0	8.26	.176
15-19 months	26.2	26.2	38.8	8.7	100.0	8.40	183
20-4 months	27.6	18.9	32.7	20.9	100.0	9.81	196
25+ months	26.9	19.4	30.6	23.1	100.0	10.68	134
Total	31.3	23.1	32.0	13.6	100.0	8.70	793

following the previous birth. The mean duration of amenorrhoea is about 9 months. It is slightly longer for births to women aged 25 or older. It does not, however, show any consistent relationship with the order of birth. It also does not vary much by sex of prior birth, or use of family planning. However, women are likely to be amenorrhoeic for a shorter duration if the previous birth did not survive, again indicating a possible effect on amenorrhoea due to the shortening of duration of breastfeeding following the death of the child.

The mean duration of amenorrhoea increases with the increase in the duration of breastfeeding. Women who breastfeed their babies for a shorter duration tend to resume ovulation relatively sooner than women who breastfeed their children longer.

5.3.5 DURATION OF POSTPARTUM ABSTINENCE

The average duration of postpartum abstinence between two live births during the five years preceding the survey is a bit longer than 5 months (Table 5.14). Older women tend to abstain from sexual relations for a somewhat longer duration following the birth of a child than younger women. The mean duration of postpartum abstinence decreases with the increase in the order of birth, but it does not vary much according to the sex of the prior birth. The custom of having the first one or two deliveries in the woman's parents' home seems to affect, to some extent, the

TABLE 5.14: SELECTED CHARACTERISTICS OF WOMEN AND SECOND- AND HIGHER-ORDER BIRTHS DURING THE FIVE YEARS PRIOR TO THE SURVEY, BY THE REPORTED DURATION OF SEXUAL ABSTINENCE FOLLOWING THE PREVIOUS BIRTH (%)

Background Characteristic	*Months Abstaining*			*Total*	*Mean*	N
	<5	*5-9*	*10+*			
Current Maternal Age						
15-19	50.8	47.8	1.5	100.0	4.31	67
20-4	46.0	43.4	10.6	100.0	5.48	376
25-9	41.2	51.3	7.5	100.0	5.24	279
30+	39.4	46.5	14.4	100.0	5.66	71
Order of Prior Birth						
1	39.3	52.1	8.7	100.0	5.48	242
2	43.2	46.5	10.4	100.0	5.46	241
3	42.1	48.3	9.7	100.0	5.31	176
4	51.2	41.9	7.0	100.0	5.14	86
5+	68.8	25.0	6.3	100.0	4.08	48
Sex of Prior Birth						
Female	42.9	48.3	8.8	100.0	5.31	387
Male	45.3	45.3	9.4	100.0	5.32	406
Survival of Prior Birth						
Still living	42.6	48.1	9.3	100.0	5.40	719
Deceased	59.5	33.8	6.8	100.0	4.50	74
Prior Pregnancy Interrupted						
Yes	36.0	54.0	10.0	100.0	5.64	50
No	44.7	46.3	9.0	100.0	5.29	743
Maternal Education						
Illiterate	46.0	44.8	9.2	100.0	5.29	574
Primary	43.4	50.9	5.7	100.0	4.96	106
Primary+	35.4	53.1	11.5	100.0	5.74	113
Use of FP Between Births						
Yes	44.1	47.1	8.8	100.0	5.74	34
No	44.1	46.8	9.1	100.0	5.30	759
Stay in Mother's House Following Prior Birth						
0 month	47.3	42.4	10.3	100.0	5.33	224
1-3 months	64.4	31.1	4.4	100.0	4.15	225
4+ months	28.8	59.9	11.3	100.0	6.07	344
Total	44.1	46.8	9.1	100.0	5.31	793

duration of postpartum abstinence. The mean duration of abstinence following a birth is slightly longer if the mother stayed at her parents' home for four months or longer than if she stayed there for less than four months.

The mean duration of postpartum abstinence is longer (8.2 months) after a sterilization, which is mostly conducted within a few months after delivery.

5.4 Timing of Sterilization

In general, sterilization marks the end of a woman's reproductive career. Of the sample of 915 women, 44 per cent were already sterilized. More Hindu women (46 per cent) have undergone sterilization than Muslim women (36 per cent).

Looking at the age pattern of women who have been sterilized, it is remarkable that of all women aged 15-19 years already 6.2 per cent are sterilized. In the age group of 25-29 the proportion is more than 60 per cent. The data indicate that at the age of 30 years old, a majority of women are sterilized. In the oldest age group of 30 plus (the oldest respondent being 42 years old), the share is more than 80 per cent, indicating the overall importance of sterilization. Also, it indicates the young ages and early stage in the reproductive career at which women bear children.

Sterilizations are mainly conducted soon after delivery: of all women who underwent a sterilization (N = 420), 47 per cent had the operation done within one month after delivery, another 30 per cent within two months and 15 per cent within 5 months.

In summary, women in the survey population marry early (15.2 years) and have their children soon after marriage. At the age of 30, more than 60 per cent of the women are already sterilized and thus have completed their reproductive career. The average duration of birth interval is 32 months. Twenty-nine per cent of the birth intervals are shorter than 24 months. The use of spacing methods hardly contributes to the duration of birth intervals, as temporary contraceptive use is very low. The most important determinants of the length of birth interval are postpartum amenorrhoea and abstinence.

6

Beliefs and Perceptions about Fertility and Child Spacing

Having described actual child spacing behaviour within the reproductive career in Chapter 5, we now turn to the second research question regarding the perceptions and beliefs of our female subjects regarding child spacing and other events in their reproductive health career. This chapter presents information on perceptions and beliefs regarding birth intervals and its proximate determinants and fertility in general. The information was collected through both survey and in-depth interviews.

Section 6.1.1 focuses on ideal family size, while Section 6.1.2 discusses the ideal sex composition of children. Section 6.2 describes the perceived duration of birth intervals (Section 6.2.1) and reasons behind such perceptions (Section 6.2.2). The proximate determinants are further examined: postpartum amenorrhoea and breastfeeding (Section 6.2.3), postpartum abstinence (Section 6.2.4), and sexual abstinence and frequency of intercourse (Section 6.2.5). In Section 6.2.6 we present the women's own views about how the ideal duration of birth intervals can be achieved.

6.1 Beliefs About Fertility

This section examines the beliefs and perceptions of women about ideal family size (Section 6.1.1) and ideal sex composition of children (Section 6.1.2).

6.1.1 Desired Number of Children

The women were asked in the survey what they thought was the ideal number of children (Table 6.1). Of all women, 932

TABLE 6.1: MEAN IDEAL NUMBER OF CHILDREN BY GENDER, ACCORDING TO HOUSEHOLD AND INDIVIDUAL BACKGROUND FACTORS

	Children Mean	N	*Sons* Mean	*Daughters* Mean	N
Household Background					
Religion					
Hindu	2.63	831	1.52	1.15	736
Muslim	2.86	90	1.65	1.24	72
Christian	2.50	2	1.50	1.00	2
Gouli tribe	3.44	9	2.11	1.33	9
Type of Family/Household					
Single					
Nuclear	2.64	315	1.53	1.15	280
Joint	2.70	318	1.57	1.18	280
Other	2.61	46	1.59	1.10	41
Co-residing					
Nuclear	2.60	168	1.52	1.13	143
Joint	2.69	75	1.53	1.20	66
Other	2.70	10	1.44	1.22	9
Individual Background					
Age group (years)					
15-19	2.85	143	1.57	1.25	130
20-4	2.59	341	1.51	1.14	299
25-9	2.67	324	1.57	1.16	285
30 +	2.59	124	1.54	1.09	105
Literacy Level					
Illiterate	2.74	735	1.59	1.18	660
Literate	2.35	197	1.33	1.08	159
Present Occupation					
Cultivation	2.71	223	1.59	1.17	200
Wage labour	2.75	297	1.56	1.18	270
Cultivation + wage labour	2.75	118	1.64	1.19	102
Household	2.51	226	1.45	1.14	191
Other	2.42	66	1.41	1.07	54
Total	2.70	932	1.54	1.16	819
According to (Opinion of Respondents)					
Husband	3.0	1.8	1.3		
Mother-in-law	3.4	1.9	1.4		
Mother	3.0	1.8	1.3		

respondents were able to give a numerical response; the average desired family size is 2.7 children. More than half (52 per cent) of the respondents consider a two-child family to be ideal and another one-third (32 per cent) consider three children to be ideal. A minority (N = 9) think that one child is enough.

Taking into account household and individual background factors, it was found that Muslim women desired 2.9 children, Hindu women 2.6. Younger women have a slightly higher figure of desired family size (2.9) than the older age groups. Illiterate women desire on average 2.8 children, literate women 2.4 children.

Focussing on the normative beliefs, as indicated in Ajzen and Fishbein's model (1980; see Chapter 2), women were asked what, in their opinion, people in their immediate environment thought would be the ideal family size. Women indicated, where important others such as mother-in-law, husband and mother were concerned, that these others had a bigger number in mind (2.7 children). It is interesting that mothers-in-law are thought to have a higher ideal family size for their daughters-in-law, i.e. 3.4 children, compared to the women's husbands or own mothers (both 3.0 children).

The women were asked in an open question *why* they desired a particular number of children. Although it turned out to be difficult to classify all the answers (sometimes more than one reason was given, for example), the answers indicate the major perceptions on desired family size.

The major reason for the desired family size is economic in character (45 per cent; see Table 6.2). Another related reason (23 per cent) is that it is difficult to take care of more children. It is worth mentioning that for some of the respondents (7 per cent), the desired number of children was linked to their ability to instil and maintain discipline in life. Health reasons play a minor role (6 per cent), as does the uncertainty of whether or not children will survive (4 per cent). Only three respondents feel that it is up to God.

One thus can conclude that the most important reasons behind the average desired family size of 2.7 children are economic in character and related to the care to be given to children. Respondents frequently indicated this in expressions such as:

TABLE 6.2: REASONS FOR DESIRING A PARTICULAR NUMBER OF CHILDREN

	%	N
1. Economic reasons: earning, work, etc.	44.6	424
2. Difficult to take care of more children	22.9	218
3. Can maintain discipline in life if number of children is small	7.4	70
4. Health reasons	5.5	52
5. No guarantee of survival	4.2	40
6. Nice to have more children	4.0	38
7. Children can keep each other company	1.9	18
8. It reduces our country's population	1.5	14
9. Up to God	0.3	3
NA	7.2	71
Total	100.0	951

It is difficult to work and earn money if there are more children.

Now the market prices are high and wages for coolie work are also low, so it is difficult to look after more than two children.

If the household does not own land it is more difficult to bring up more children:

There is no family farm and property. It is difficult to work and earn money if there are more children.

Often an implicit comparison of the present expensive situation with the past is made:

In these costly days and limited income, we can manage only three children.

The desire to have a limited number of children is related to the costs of food, education and clothes, and the necessity to care for them and give them affection:

We can provide all facilities like education, good food and clothing if there are only three children.

and

If there are more than two, they cannot get love and affection and they will quarrel.

Very few respondents mentioned the reverse relationship, i.e.

wanting to have more children so that they can later earn money, thus adding to the family income. These findings provide solid backing for Caldwell's (1976 and 1982) theory on the reverse flow of wealth: instead of children having to take care of the earnings of the family, parents have to provide care to the children. The quality of children obviously plays a role: children should be fed, clothed and educated, and they need love and affection.

Other reasons play only minor roles. Respondents (6 per cent) cited health factors, either their own health or that of their children:

> If I have more than two children, I will become weak and lose energy.

and

> If there are only two children, they will be healthy.

Child survival plays a minor role: only a few respondents (5.5 per cent) said that because of their uncertainty that all their children will survive, a bigger family size seems sensible:

> If something happens to one child the other two will survive, so it is good to have three children.

In this the survival of sons plays a major role (see Section 6.1.2).

Some respondents said that they prefer an even number of children (sons or daughters), as they can keep each other company. Fourteen respondents pointed out that the population policy of the Indian government was a reason to have a certain desired family size:

> As per government rules we should not have more children.

Only a few respondents (N = 3) said that the number of children they get is up to God:

> Whatever the number might be, it is in God's hand.

The influence of the social environment on desired family size becomes clear in the following statement:

> If we have only one child, people will tease.

In summary, this section sketches the 'fertility context' of the research area as one where people do not want to have as many

children as possible: on average the respondents wanted only 2.7 children. The reasons for this are mainly economic in character: parents have to provide food, clothing and education to the children, which are considered to be costly. We can relate these findings to the theory of Caldwell (1976 and 1982) on the flow of wealth.

The survival of children still plays a role: some people want to have more children to make sure that enough children survive, especially sons as will be seen later. It is interesting to note that respondents think that important others, and especially their mother-in-law want them to have more children than they themselves want.

6.1.2 DESIRED NUMBER OF SONS AND DAUGHTERS

Similarly, women were asked what, according to them, is the ideal sex composition of a family, i.e. the ideal number of sons and daughters (see also Table 6.1). An average of 1.5 sons and 1.2 daughters is considered to be ideal. Of all respondents, 44 per cent preferred to have only one son, another 41 per cent two sons. Of all women, 73 per cent considered only one daughter to be ideal. It is important to note that only one per cent of all women (N = 8) do not want to have a daughter at all. Two daughters are wanted by 15 per cent. The data thus clearly indicate that women do not only want sons, but many want at least one daughter. To quote a respondent:

> It is nice to have children of both sexes.

Rather exceptional are the two women who said that they do not want to have any son. Still 13 per cent of women had no preference for either sex of the child. This is typically expressed as:

> Children are children (whether male or female).

Again, when asked about the normative beliefs, respondents indicated they think important others (mother-in-law, husband, mother) want them to have a higher number of sons, as compared to their own view about the number of boys.

When women were asked about the major reason for desiring

TABLE 6.3: REASONS FOR DESIRING A PARTICULAR NUMBER OF SONS

	%	N
1. Boy will earn and work	26.3	250
2. Boy will look after parents	19.7	187
2. Boy will continue family name or property remains in the family	7.7	73
4. Boy will earn and carry the dead body	7.4	70
5. Boy will help his father and show him affection	7.4	70
6. Boy lights the lamp in the house	6.2	59
7. It is good to have an equal number of children or boys can keep each other company	2.7	26
8. People will tease if there is no male child	2.3	22
9. Everyone prefers a boy, it is the trend nowadays	1.3	12
10. If there is a son, daughter-in-law joins the family	1.1	10
11. Boy shows affection to his sister	0.6	6
12. All are the same, no sex preference	8.3	79
13. If we prefer a certain sex, we will get more children	0.4	4
14. Up to God	1.4	13
15. Other	0.2	2
NA	7.1	68
Total	100.0	951

a certain number of sons (see Table 6.3), more than one-quarter (26 per cent) related it to the fact that boys can earn and work and thus support the family. Another 20 per cent of women said that the boy will look after the parents. Another 8 per cent said that a boy will continue the family name and keep the family property, while 7 per cent felt that a boy will earn money and carry the dead body of the parents. Another 7 per cent said that boys are especially for the sake of the father, as they would show affection to their father, while 6 per cent indicated that a boy will light the lamp in the house:

A boy will continue our family and he is *kuladeepa* for our family.

Kuladeepa means family's (*kula*) lamp or light. Traditionally each family has a light or lamp lit in front of their family God. The lamp is supposed to be lighted all the time. The son of the family inherits the light and is supposed to ensure that the lamp stays lighted, i.e. to continue the family line. Also, the son here is compared to the light that symbolizes spiritual guidance, i.e. the

son is the person who shows the path of heaven to his ancestors.

A reason for wanting 2 or 4 sons is that they will keep each other company for life (3 per cent).

The strong influence of the social environment and possible consequences of not having a son become clear in the following statement:

> If a woman does not have at least one male child, the elders in their house decide to arrange a second marriage.

The interviews among men revealed the social pressure put on men as well. Friends and other people in the village pass comments such as:

> No male children to this *sulimaga* . . . fathered only female children . . . his life is not worth living.

and

> *Che!* He doesn't have a male issue. Difficult in old age!

When women were asked why they desired a particular number of daughters (see Table 6.4), the major reason mentioned is that girls will help in the household (20 per cent). More specifically, girls will help the mother. This does not only include household work, a girl is also considered to be emotionally closer to her mother, and to provide care to her:

> To help mothers in household work and to share feelings, a girl is needed.

and

> The mother's life will be fulfilled by having a female child.

Sometimes girls are considered to actually take more care of their parents (6 per cent) than sons would:

> Parents think that the son can look after them in old age and sometimes he may not look after the parents, then a girl will definitely do so.

and

> A male is required to continue our family and they will be looking after our property, but really speaking, only girls do take care of parents.

Also, in general, girls are considered to be more affectionate:

> Girls are more affectionate than boys. So there should be two girls and one

TABLE 6.4: REASONS FOR DESIRING A PARTICULAR NUMBER OF DAUGHTERS

	%	N
1. Girl helps in the household	20.4	194
2. 'Girl looks nice in the house'	14.7	140
3. Girl cries when we die	12.7	121
4. A girl is for another family	10.1	96
5. Girl shows affection to parents	5.6	53
6. Girl 'goes and comes' to husbands' and parents' place	5.0	48
7. Girl will look after parents during illness or in old age	2.6	25
8. If there is no girl, people will tease	2.5	24
9. It is good to have an equal number of girls	2.0	19
10. Girl is for *aarti*	1.8	17
11. There should be only one girl, otherwise it will be difficult to give dowry	1.5	14
12. Up to God	1.5	14
13. Girl decorates our body after we die	1.3	12
14. Girl shows affection to her brother	0.5	5
15. All are the same, no sex preference	8.2	78
16. If we prefer a certain sex of the child, we will get more children	0.6	6
17. If there is no girl, there are no problems	0.8	8
NA	8.1	77
Total	100.0	951

boy. A boy may or may not look after the parents, but a girl will definitely look after the parents in their old age.

The care and emotional attachment that daughters have is further illustrated by the statement, mentioned by almost 13 per cent of the respondents, that when the parents die, it is the girl who will cry:

> Boys carry the body on their shoulders, but when we die the daughters cry.

A mere one per cent of the women stated, relating to a Kannada proverb, that a girl is needed to decorate the body of the parents.

Another 15 per cent of the respondents said that 'a girl in the house looks nice (*chand*)'. Women say that a girl is for the sake of *aarti* (2 per cent). *Aarti* is the ceremony of waving the lights, only

to be conducted by women. One respondent relates the role of daughters to the role of sons:

For *aarti* sake a girl is necessary, for *keerati* sake a boy is needed.

Keerati literally means honour or fame: the son is supposed to bring honour and fame to the family. In other words, a family without a son vanishes unheard of. Other respondents mentioned:

A girl is Laxmi (Laxmi is the goddess of wealth and richness).

Only 1.5 per cent of the women related the desired number of girls to difficulties in providing a dowry:

We can not manage the marriage expenses of girls.

Some women (5 per cent) responded that they actually like it that daughters after their marriage and having moved to their husband's house, will continue to visit their parents' house (in local language: 'coming and going'):

Female children are attractive to our house. After the girl is married she visits her mother's place, it is nice for us.

Again, the influence of the social environment plays a role as indicated by 2.5 per cent of the respondents: people will tease if a family does not have a girl.

6.2 Beliefs About Spacing

Questions about women's beliefs and perceptions about child spacing were also posed in the survey. Open questions focused on the perceived ideal duration of birth intervals (Section 6.2.1) and the reasons behind such perception (Section 6.2.2). Section 6.2.3 discusses the proximate determinants of postpartum amenorrhoea and breastfeeding while postpartum abstinence is presented in Section 6.2.4 and sexual abstinence and frequency of intercourse in general in Section 6.2.5. Section 6.2.6 in addition focuses on the ideas of respondents themselves about how to achieve the reported ideal duration of birth intervals.

6.2.1 Ideal Duration of Birth Intervals

All women were asked about the ideal duration between marriage and first birth and between two subsequent births. Only,919 and

928 women, respectively, were able to give numerical responses to these two questions. Table 6.5 indicates the mean ideal duration according to selected household and individual background characteristics of the respondents. In total, respondents considered 31 months to be the ideal duration between marriage and first birth, and 36 months as the ideal duration between two consecutive births. It should be noted that the average duration of actual birth intervals is 32 months (see Chapter 5).

TABLE 6.5: MEAN IDEAL DURATION OF FIRST AND HIGHER ORDER BIRTH INTERVALS BY HOUSEHOLD AND INDIVIDUAL BACKGROUND

	First Birth Interval		*Higher Order Birth Intervals*	
	Mean	N	*Mean*	N
Household Background				
Religion				
Hindu	31.6	819	36.0	826
Muslim	29.1	89	36.5	91
Christian	36.0	2	48.0	2
Gouli tribe	34.7	9	33.3	9
Type of Family/Household				
Single				
Nuclear	31.0	307	36.6	313
Joint	31.2	316	36.1	315
Other	31.1	47	34.7	46
Co-residing				
Nuclear	32.3	167	35.3	172
Joint	31.2	72	36.2	72
Other	37.2	10	34.8	10
Individual Background				
Age Group (years)				
15-19	28.6	144	34.3	142
20-4	31.0	332	35.5	337
25-9	32.0	321	36.4	324
30+	34.1	122	38.4	125
Literacy Level				
Illiterate	31.3	722	35.5	731
Literate	31.8	197	38.0	197

Contd.

TABLE 6.5 (Contd.)

	First Birth Interval		*Higher Order Birth Intervals*	
	Mean	N	*Mean*	N
Present Occupation				
Cultivation	33.0	217	35.6	221
Wage labour	30.8	293	35.1	294
Cultivation + wage labour	30.9	118	35.4	119
Household	30.5	224	36.9	226
Other	32.1	66	36.0	66
Total	31.4	919	36.0	928
According to				
Husband	NA		33.8	523
Mother-in-law	NA		31.9	409
Mother	NA		33.3	568

Less than half of the women (43 per cent) considered 24 months as the ideal duration between marriage and first birth, 29 per cent preferred a duration of 36 months, whereas only 9 per cent of them felt that the first birth should occur within 23 months after marriage. With respect to the ideal interval between two consecutive births, 27 per cent of the women preferred to have a gap of 24 months, and 46 per cent a gap of 36 months. Only 1 per cent of the women thought that the next birth should occur within 23 months after the previous birth.

Only very small differences were observed among women living in different kinds of families and households. Muslims considered a slightly shorter first birth interval to be ideal (29 months against 32 months for Hindus and 34 months for Gouli women). Regarding the interval between two consecutive births, Muslims considered the ideal duration to be 37 months, just one month longer than Hindus (36 months).

Women who are younger than 19 years preferred 29 months between marriage and birth of the first child and 34 months between two births. Both mean values increase with the increase in age of women: women beyond 30 years preferred 35 months and 38 months, respectively, for first and consecutive birth interval.

The influence of a woman's education on ideal duration is found to vary both in case of first birth and between two births.

However the mean ideal duration between marriage and first birth and between two births is greater for women with higher than primary-level education than for women who are less educated. The mean ideal duration between marriage and first birth and between two births stays more or less constant at 31-32 months and 36 months respectively for different levels of husband's education.

In addition, the women were asked what—in their view—important others feel is the ideal birth interval between two consecutive births for them. According to our respondents, their mothers-in-law considered the mean ideal birth interval to be 31.9 months, which is considerably shorter than their own ideal of 36 months. Also their husbands and their own mothers are thought to consider a slightly shorter birth interval to be ideal for them, i.e. 33.8 months and 33.3 months, respectively.

The results clearly indicate that women themselves are very well aware that a longer interval is better. The ideal (mean) durations are not very different from the actual (mean) duration of birth intervals, i.e. 32 months and 36 months respectively.

6.2.2 REASONS BEHIND IDEAL DURATION OF FIRST BIRTH INTERVAL

Respondents were asked why they consider this particular interval to be ideal. During the fieldwork, it turned out that respondents often adopted a different time perspective. Many of them for example started their explanation with 'there should be some distance (*sulp dur agati*)' or 'It is good to be a bit late (*sulp tada chello aiti*)'.

Also, on asking women in the in-depth interviews when their first child was born after marriage, a typical answer was that it was born within one year after marriage. The wording 'within one year after marriage' does not necessarily indicate the actual timing, but that it happened soon after marriage. Additionally, quite a number of respondents indicated that the first child was born late, by which it meant a period of 3 years or more.

Table 6.6 reports the different reasons, as given by the respondents, for the ideal duration of the first birth interval. Of all women, 21 per cent said that the reported ideal duration is good for the health of the woman:

TABLE 6.6: REASONS FOR A PARTICULAR DURATION OF IDEAL FIRST BIRTH INTERVAL (SURVEY)

	%	N
1. Good for woman's health	20.8	198
2. Women are young when they marry	15.6	148
3. If too early or if too late, people will tease	13.9	132
4. Husband and wife get to know each other or live happily together or stay free of commitments	10.1	96
5. Knowledge about having children	7.8	74
6. Time to visit (go and come) parents' place	7.3	69
7. Time to move freely around	7.0	67
8. Troublesome to women if too early or too late	3.4	32
9. Working in husband's house	2.7	26
10. 'Playing child will have a troubling infant' (*aduva makkalige kaduva kusu)*	2.5	24
10. Wants children as soon as possible	1.9	18
12. Up to God	1.4	13
13. Others	0.3	3
NA	5.2	51
Total	100.0	951

It leads to good health for the woman, she could earn some income, she could eat certain foods which gives her strength.

Women use particular expressions to indicate poor health:

As the woman is young at the time of marriage, her waist is not strong. After three years she will become strong.

and a respondent who got her child too early indicates the negative effects on her health:

Now all bones in my body are lose.

Of all respondents, 16 per cent related an ideal duration between marriage and birth of the first child to the young age at time of marriage. Three per cent of the respondents said that women will have problems when they get children soon after marriage:

We are young at the time of our marriage, and it is not good for our health if we give birth to a child early.

and

If she gets a child earlier (than two years after marriage) she looks older for her age.

The negative effect of having a child too soon after marriage is aptly expressed by a Kannada proverb which was quoted in the responses of 3 per cent of the respondents:

> People will tease as *playing child has got a crying baby* if the couple is young and they have a child.

Of the respondents, 8 per cent say that women should first obtain some knowledge before having children:

> After four years is good. The woman will be strong and healthy and can understand the responsibilities of motherhood.

The strong influence of the social environment (mentioned by 14 per cent) is evident in the teasing that goes on in instances of young couples having a child too 'early':

> If the first birth is early people will tease, and if the gap between the children is longer than is usual then also people will tease.

and

> People will tease: '*she came with the child*' if she gets a child within two years.

Elders are usually happy when the first pregnancy and childbirth take place soon after marriage:

> for us it is good as long as there is a gap. But the elders start worrying after two years if she has not yet conceived. They say even after two years of marriage she has not got children.

Sometimes, if a woman does not give birth to a child in due time there can be severe consequences:

> My husband himself wanted to have a second marriage because my first child was born after two years of marriage.

Another 10 per cent of the respondents indicated that husband and wife should have enough time after marriage to get to know each other. Seven per cent said that there should be some freedom to move around. Another 7 per cent indicated the importance of newly-married women being able to travel to their parents' place, thus easing the process of adaptation in her husband's place. Some time between marriage and first birth is considered to be good not only for the woman, but also for the couple:

Both husband and wife can live happily together (if interval is two years).

and

Love between husband and wife will decrease if they get early issue.

Three per cent of the respondents indicated that it was good to have a longer first birth interval so that they could work and earn some money first:

I delivered the first child by the end of second year. . . . I had to stop working and so I stopped earning. I felt it was early. In our house there were only two of us (husband and wife). We had to earn and eat. There was no one else in the house to take care of. So I felt that it would have been better it I had conceived late. I could have worked and earned for two more years. When the children are very young, we have to be at home, without going for work.

One and a half per cent of the women said that the duration of the interval between marriage and birth of the first child is up to God:

It is up to God, it is not in our hands.

and

It is fate. It is not in our control. . . .

It was interesting to note that the two higher educated respondents who married at a later age had their first child within one year after marriage. The two case studies reflect the general trend of educated Indian women marrying later but having their first child soon after marriage, as well as the social norm on age at motherhood:

It would have been better if there was a gap of one more year or two more years. But we didn't use anything. So, that was very early. If it was a little late, we could have been comfortable to some extent and we could go to some place. If marriage takes place at an early age, then conception may be late. But I was 21. That is the proper age for getting children.

Another finding revealed a perception about fecundity in the first birth interval as expressed by a mother-in-law:

It is better for them if they have their first child a little late. But if they marry 4-5 years after menarche, their body would have heat (*kaavu*) inside. So they conceive soon.

The case study suggests that after menarche, heat is believed to build up in the body. After 4-5 years, enough heat is created and conception is easier than at the time of menarche. This can be clearly related to some of the biomedical studies mentioned in Chapter 2 which report on long periods of adolescents' sub-fecundity (Nair, 1993; Foster et al., 1986), i.e. anovulatory cycles occurring after menarche. The concept of heat (*kaavu*) will be explained later in Chapter 8.

6.2.3 REASONS BEHIND IDEAL DURATION OF CONSECUTIVE BIRTH INTERVALS

Table 6.7 indicates the reasons of women for the ideal birth interval between two consecutive births. More than 40 per cent of the respondents related birth interval to the stage of development of the elder child:

Three years is good, the previous child would have *grown and would eats by himself*. So it will be easy for the mother to look after the new-born baby.

and

Two years is good, the child is able to *walk independently*.

and

Three years is good, as they can *eat with their own hands*.

TABLE 6.7: REASONS FOR A PARTICULAR DURATION OF IDEAL BIRTH INTERVAL

	%	N
1. Older child eat by his own hand, can walk, play, etc.	41.3	393
2. Health of the previous child	18.0	171
3. Difficult to look after both children or elders	17.7	168
4. Health of mother and children	7.2	68
5. Health of both children	6.1	58
6. Health of mother	4.2	40
7. If no breastmilk, or insufficient, child cannot be breastfed properly	1.8	17
8. Other reasons	0.8	8
NA	2.9	28
Total	100.0	951

and

> Three years is good because the previous child will *move around by itself*, so it is easy for me.

and

> Two years is good, the first child grows and then it *plays by itself*.

and

> Two years is good, they can walk and attend to their *natural call*.

Another 18 per cent of the women indicated that a particular duration of birth interval would be better for the health of the older child:

> If the gap is three years the previous child one will grow nicely.

and

> The first child will not get sufficient milk if is it early (earlier than three years).

Another 7 per cent related the ideal duration to the health of both children:

> If we keep a gap between the children their health will be good; otherwise they will become weak.

while almost 18 per cent said that it would be difficult to look after both children if the interval is too short:

> Three years is good . . . both children will get the affection of the mother.

Seven per cent of the respondents related the duration of birth intervals to the health of their children and their own health:

> Two years is good as both mother and child will be in good health and mother will gain strength in her waist.

Only 4 per cent of the respondents related the ideal duration to their own health. A few women related the ideal interval to the fact that they have to work:

> Most of the women have to work outside so it is difficult to leave the small child in the house and go to work. So a duration of three years is needed so that the child will grow up.

6.2.4 IDEAL DURATION OF POSTPARTUM AMENORRHOEA AND BREASTFEEDING

Women were also asked about the ideal duration of the proximate determinants of postpartum amenorrhoea, breastfeeding and postpartum abstinence. Of the total number of respondents, 906 (amenorrhoea), 930 (breastfeeding) and 907 (abstinence) were able to provide numerical responses. Table 6.8 shows the mean ideal duration of these determinants according to household and individual background characteristics.

Women in general considered 11.7 months to be the mean ideal duration for postpartum amenorrhoea. Slightly less than half of them (43 per cent) preferred 12 months' duration, 15 per cent a 24 month-duration and almost one-fourth (24 per cent) considered less than 6 months as the ideal duration. Note that the actual duration of postpartum amenorrhoea is 9 months (see Chapter 5).

Some women said they preferred a short duration of postpartum amenorrhoea, as menstruation would 'remove the dirt from the stomach':

> Unwanted dirty things will go out of the stomach.

Similar ideas about menstruation cleaning the stomach are described in Chapter 8.

The mean ideal duration of postpartum amenorrhoea increases with age. Not much variation is found in differing levels of respondent's education.

With regard to breastfeeding, the respondents believed that the child should be breastfed, on average, for about 18 months. Almost 40 per cent preferred a duration of 12 months, whereas 31 per cent considered a duration of 24 months ideal. Only 7 per cent of the women preferred to breastfeed less than one year.

Differences in religion and ethnicity can be observed (although the number of Christians and Gouli are limited): Gouli women consider 23.3 months as the ideal period to breastfeed. The two Christian women think that one year is enough, while Hindus and Muslims do not differ much. Younger women prefer a slightly longer duration of breastfeeding than older women.

In addition, women were asked whether they know the reasons

TABLE 6.8: MEAN IDEAL DURATION OF POSTPARTUM AMENORRHOEA, BREASTFEEDING AND POSTPARTUM ABSTINENCE, ACCORDING TO HOUSEHOLD AND INDIVIDUAL BACKGROUND

	Postpartum Amenorrhoea		*Breast-feeding*		*Postpartum Abstinence*	
	Mean	*N*	*Mean*	*N*	*Mean*	*N*
Household Background						
Religion						
Hindu	11.7	806	18.0	828	8.5	807
Muslim	11.7	89	17.5	91	5.9	89
Christian	15.0	2	12.0	2	8.5	2
Gouli tribe	13.7	9	23.3	9	5.8	9
Type of Family/ Household						
Single						
Nuclear	12.2	306	17.8	313	8.0	304
Joint	11.2	309	17.9	317	8.3	309
Other	10.5	45	17.2	46	6.7	44
Co-residing						
Nuclear	12.3	164	18.3	170	8.2	167
Joint	12.1	72	19.4	74	9.4	73
Other	7.4	10	20.4	10	7.3	10
Individual Background						
Age Group (years)						
15-19	10.8	143	18.8	145	7.5	139
20-4	11.8	330	18.2	335	7.9	333
25-9	11.8	311	17.6	325	8.7	315
30+	2.3	122	17.8	125	8.6	120
Literacy Level						
Illiterate	11.6	714	18.0	733	8.3	711
Literate	12.0	192	18.1	197	7.9	196
Present Occupation						
Cultivation	11.4	217	18.3	222	8.4	215
Wage labour	12.6	293	17.8	294	8.7	288
Cultivation+ wage labour	10.9	118	18.0	119	7.9	117
Household	11.3	224	17.7	227	7.6	220
Other	11.7	66	18.4	66	7.4	66
Total	11.7	906	18.0	930	8.2	907

for postpartum amenorrhoea (*muttu illa*, not having a menstruation), i.e. whether they know that it is determined by the frequency and duration of breastfeeding (see Table 6.9). Most women (82 per cent) do not know the reason for postpartum amenorrhoea. Another 15 per cent mentioned another reason: because women loose a lot of blood during delivery, no blood is left in their bodies for menstruation. It takes time to regain the blood, i.e. the duration of postpartum amenorrhoea:

> More blood is lost at the time of delivery. It has to be recollected.

Others added that women are weak after delivery, and the condition of being weak and having less blood is interrelated (see Chapter 8). The duration of postpartum amenorrhoea then depends on the health of women: the weaker they are, the longer the period lasts:

> Much of the blood is lost at the time of delivery and a woman becomes weak. If she takes good food regularly then her periods will start early, otherwise it will be late.

and

> During delivery, blood is lost, so periods may be delayed. If the delivery is in hospital, they may give tablets and tonics so the time of not having periods will be shorter. If the delivery occurs at home, the time of not having periods will be longer.

Various kinds of reasoning illustrated in Table 6.9 might provide an insight into the question following Chapter 5: how are women in the research area able to achieve an average birth interval of 32 months when they hardly use any spacing methods? In Chapter 5 we concluded that postpartum amenorrhoea, induced by breastfeeding, and postpartum abstinence seem to be the most

TABLE 6.9: KNOWING REASONS FOR DURATION OF POSTPARTUM AMENORRHOEA?

	%	*N*
No	81.7	777
Yes, but other reason	15.0	143
Up to God	1.1	10
Yes, related to breastfeeding	0.3	3
NA	1.9	18

important determinants of the length of birth intervals. The perceived reason for postpartum amenorrhoea suggests an additional link, i.e. postpartum amenorrhoea related to the nutritional status of a woman. In Chapter 2, we learnt of a study by Ford and Kim (1993) in Bangladesh which indicates that nutritional status of women can indeed determine the duration of postpartum infecundability: among women weighing more than 44 kg the duration of postpartum amenorrhoea was 13.6 months, among women weighing less than 38 kg the duration was 17.6 months.

6.2.5 IDEAL DURATION OF POSTPARTUM ABSTINENCE

In the local language Kannada, different words and concepts are used to indicate sexual relations: *hasege maartaare* (literally: making the bed), sitting together (*kuditaare* or *kududu*) or *prapancha* (literally: the world). Sexual abstinence is indicated with the word *hasege pathya,* literally meaning abstinence from the bed. It is also referred to as *dur irbeeku* (there should be some distance between husband and wife).

Women in the survey were asked about their view of the ideal duration of postpartum abstinence (*hasege pathya* in Kannada). The mean ideal duration of postpartum abstinence amounts to 8.2 months. About 20 per cent of the women preferred to have a mean duration of abstinence of 5 months, 22 per cent of 6 months and 27 per cent of 12 months. One-third of the women preferred a duration of less than 6 months.

Both Muslim and Gouli women preferred a short duration of postpartum abstinence (5.9 and 5.8 months respectively) while Hindus and Christian women preferred a period of 8.5 months. Women living in joint families, either single or co-residing, wanted a slightly longer duration of postpartum abstinence (8.3 and 9.4 months, respectively) than women living in nuclear, either single or co-residing, families (8.0 and 8.2 months respectively). Also, older women preferred a longer duration of postpartum abstinence than younger women, while literate women wanted a slightly shorter duration (7.9 months) than illiterate women (8.3 months). Note that the actual duration of postpartum abstinence is five months (see Chapter 5).

Chapter 5 indicates a clear link between the duration of postpartum abstinence and the custom of staying in mother's place (*tavaru mane*) during and after delivery. Women who stayed in their mother's place after delivery refrained longer from sexual contacts (6 months) than women who stayed in their husband's house (5.3 months). Women who returned from their mother's place to their husband's house within there months after delivery had the shortest duration of postpartum abstinence, i.e. 4.2 months. As described by a respondent in an in-depth interview:

> Even after delivery if we come to husband's house early, then again it starts early. If we come after five months, conception also will be late by that amount of time. It depends upon how we observe it.

According to the female respondents, usually the women are told to observe *hasege pathya* after delivery, by either their mother-in-law, elders, or mother:

> They tell us (women) . . . the mother-in-law or the grandmother. But we have to understand ourselves and follow it. We have to tell our husbands. If they listen to us it is good. If they don't listen to us, what can we do?

and

> Mother tells this. Mother-in-law usually doesn't talk about it. In *tavaru mane* mother herself tells this. Such things cannot be told (in husband's place). They feel ashamed to tell it. They hope that the couple has that knowledge and follows it.

On asking the reason behind the custom of postpartum abstinence, respondents attributed it, like they do for many other customs, in the following way:

> It is followed by the elders,

thereby indicating that they follow the elder's advices, while they themselves do not know much about the reason:

> . . . why they started such a custom, I don't know.

A few women expressed their opinion as follows:

> It is better if she stays for five months in *tavaru mane*. The child will grow a little and conception will also be late. Perhaps it is for that reason that they have formed such a custom. It is not good during *hasi may* (vulnerable period after delivery)

and

> With the intention of keeping our body healthy, we have to take such care.

In the in-depth interviews among men, respondents indicated that sexual intercourse should be avoided after delivery because women are in *hasi may* and that

> It is painful for women.

They also described more specific consequences such as:

> *Gantu irtaiti* (a knot will be there) . . . *nanju agtaiti* (tetanus or sepsis will occur), *mai allagirtaiti* (her body will be like puffed up rice)

and

> As the body becomes loose after delivery, elders have made a rule that she should not have sex until her body become tight.

On asking what would happen if a woman becomes pregnant soon after delivery, thus indicating that the couple did not observe *hasege pathya*, a female respondent explained:

> People blame them for that because it is not good . . . that it is not good to become pregnant so early. People blame their elders also that they should have told them about it.

Another respondent added:

> The woman will suffer from a disease which is found especially among women who have just delivered. . . . In our village, there was a woman who had to go to husband's house two months after the delivery, because there was nobody to work in the house. But soon her body had a severe swelling. Then she was admitted to the hospital and recovered slowly.

The respondents however did not think that everyone really complies with the rule:

> Many people don't follow it. Only 10 per cent of people follow this custom. More people don't follow it.

and

> It is difficult. These days nobody will be ready to follow it. Maybe one in ten men follow it. Perhaps in the olden days people listened.

Indeed, a mother-in-law, comparing the past with the present, said that in earlier times, postpartum abstinence was followed

for a longer time, thus leading to longer birth intervals:

In the past, elders used to tell and the younger used to obey. They did not have sex for one or one-and-half years. So there was a gap of three to four years between two children. . . . Elders used to tell and the younger people used to obey. But now nobody listens to the elders. They decide everything themselves, get two or three children and then get operated.

6.2.6 PERCEPTIONS ABOUT SEXUAL ABSTINENCE AND FREQUENCY OF INTERCOURSE

Besides postpartum abstinence, sexual abstinence can also affect the duration of birth intervals (see Chapter 2). Information on sexual abstinence as related to other reproductive events (rather than birth and delivery), to religious or festival days and periodic abstinence was gathered through survey and in-depth interviews. Sexual abstinence appears to be quite prevalent in Indian society.

(a) Sexual Abstinence Related to Other Reproductive Events

The practice of sexual abstinence is quite prevalent in Indian society. It is not only in force in the postpartum period, but also during other stages in the reproductive career: after an abortion, during menstruation, during pregnancy and after sterilization.

After the abortion it is usually followed. Usually it is practised for one month.

and

. . . We follow the *hasege pathya* during the five days when we have M.C.

and

My mother-in-law was telling how to take care, etc., during pregnancy. We also used to be careful. She had told that up to four months we should not have sexual relationship (*prapancha*).

and

After the operation it is advised to abstain for six months. Some may follow it and some may not. But it is good if we follow it. They advise in the hospital. . . . For eight months to one year.

and

. . . After the current operation (laparoscopy) abstinence is advised for three months and after *holige* operation (tubectomy) it is advised for six months.

Men indicated that *hasege pathya* should be observed about 5-6 days during menstruation because

That is dirty ... blood infects.

and

Because children will be born.

or

Child born will not be well . . . it will be crippled or will have some disease (*muttu dosha*).

The last two perceptions indicate that men think that the fertile period is at the time of menstruation.

Like postpartum abstinence, refraining from sexual contact is mainly related to the health of women:

They (hospital) had told us everything, even *hasege pathya*. We had to follow everything for about a year . . . also *hasege pathya*. . . . For one year. We followed all the advice. We followed it in the interest of our health.

A respondent estimated that:

75 per cent of men don't follow it. Only 25 per cent of people follow, because they have some knowledge.

(b) Sexual Abstinence Related to Religious Days or Festivals, or Other Reasons

The survey revealed that there were several religious festivals, as reported by both female and male respondents, during which couples should not engage in sexual relationships. Some women mentioned all festivals, some only the big festivals (*dodda habba*), while others were more specific about the number of days during certain festivals on which one should refrain from sexual relations.

On death anniversaries of ancestors, all *puja* (worship) days, and days with religious functions, one should abstain from sex.

Several respondents mentioned all full-moon (*hunnime*) and new-moon (*amawasya*) days, while others mentioned specific full- and new-moon days in certain months of the year. Also at the time of a lunar or solar eclipse one should avoid having sex.

Other respondents mentioned Tuesdays and Fridays, sometimes in specific months, as days on which they abstain from sexual contact. Others mentioned special days in the week on which sexual relations should be avoided. For example, couples avoid sex every Saturday or every Friday and Monday.

Also some women said that they abstained from sex when the house is cleaned or the beds are washed, or when there is a fair. Another respondent mentioned that couples should refrain from sex when the children become older.

Newly-wed couples are not supposed to have sexual relations in the so-called bad months (*ketta tingla* in Kannada or *karab mina* in Urdu) during the first year of their marriage (period covering December–January, July–August).

Abstinence from sexual relations for religious reasons is attributed to the fact that sexual relationships are polluting and one can not approach the Gods (or provide food to them) while in a polluted state (see also Chapter 8). A big difference with sexual abstinence observed after reproductive events, as mentioned above, is the consequence of not obeying the rules. If *hasege pathya* is not observed as it is related to religious functions, something bad will happen to the family and the household (disputes or illness). Respondents therefore believe that people are more eager and willing to observe sexual abstinence during religious days than after reproductive events.

For a more detailed overview, refer to Hutter, et al. (2002).

(c) Periodic Abstinence

Periodic abstinence is hardly practised in the research area: only 6 out of 951 respondents in the survey knew about the method. Those who claimed to know the method were not always able to identify fecund and not-fecund phases in the menstrual cycle. However, while explaining the method, many a respondent showed interest about knowing more about the method.

(d) Frequency of Intercourse

The interviews among men indicated that frequency of sexual intercourse is very high during the first year of marriage and that the frequency reduces after the birth of a child. The frequency reduces still further after the birth of subsequent children. Also women said that their sexual relationship changed over the life course:

> In the beginning of married life they (couple) will have a separate room. Then after having children and with increasing age it changes. In old age both of them sleep in different places. . . . After some years they stop having sex. Then till the children are young, they sleep together. When they (children) reach the age of understanding every thing, then the parents stop sleeping together. . . . After they get daughters and son-in-law they think that these people may laugh at them if they continue to have such a relationship. So they stop then.

A general conception is indeed that once a woman is a grandmother she should stop having sex. Note that in the context of a village a woman can be a grandmother at the age of 30-35 years.

Almost all men related sexual intercourse (and loss of semen) to loss of energy. Most felt that it is difficult for labourers to have frequent sex: they do not have enough food to eat and cannot regain the strength that is lost during sex. If one keeps away from sex, the body remains solid and healthy:

> The man who used to lift a bag full of paddy before, will not be able to do it after sex.

and

> The fat man becomes thin due to too much of sex.

This loss of energy is referred to *dhat(u)*, i.e. symptoms related to the loss of semen. Respondents also say:

> Man becomes hollow (*pollu*) if he has sex daily.

and

> It is not good to have sex daily, or frequently. It is okay to have sex once a week, or once in 15 days or once in a month. . . .

Sexual intercourse is considered to heat up the body (see further Chapter 8).

Although men say that sexual intercourse will not affect their wife's energy, women indicated in the interviews that for them as well sexual intercourse means loss of energy. The reasoning, however, seems to be more related to the risk of becoming pregnant again (leading to loss of energy):

> It is good if we have it fewer times. . . . Because it is said that the strength will be lost if they have relations too often. It will be better if we live separately as far as possible (*dur irbeeku*). But a man may ask, 'Why have we married you? To stay away from you?' Then if we convince them at that time, they understand in a better way. For men there will be no problem. But women have problems . . . the problems of delivery and of the monthly menstruation. Men don't have such problems.

6.2.7 HOW TO ACHIEVE IDEAL DURATION OF BIRTH INTERVALS?

After having asked about the ideal duration of birth intervals and the proximate determinants, the women were subsequently asked how they could achieve this ideal duration (see Table 6.10). More

TABLE 6.10: METHODS THAT CAN BE USED TO ACHIEVE IDEAL BIRTH INTERVAL, ACCORDING TO RESPONDENTS

	%	N
1. I do not know	41.3	393
2. Copper-T or oral pill	15.6	148
3. Oral pill	12.0	114
4. Copper-T	6.4	61
5. Abstinence	4.9	47
6. It is up to God	3.4	32
7. Modern and traditional methods	3.2	30
8. Oral pill, tablets for induced abortion + abstinence	2.8	27
9. Copper-T or condom	2.3	22
10. Copper-T or induced abortion	1.5	14
11. Oral pill or Copper-T + injection	1.2	11
12. Oral pill or condom	0.8	8
12. Condom	0.2	2
NA	2.3	22
Total	100.0	951

than 40 per cent did not know how to achieve what they found to be the ideal duration. Almost one-third of the respondents talked about the oral pill, followed by a slightly lower proportion of respondents mentioning Copper-T (more than one method could be mentioned). Only a few women reported condoms. In addition, almost 8 per cent stated abstinence from sexual relationships, 4 per cent induced abortion. Three and a half per cent of the respondents said that God decides on the duration of birth interval.

A total of about 48 per cent of women reported the use of oral pill, Copper-T, condom, induced abortion, abortion tablets or traditional methods to achieve the ideal duration of birth interval. However, Chapter 5 already indicated that women hardly use any spacing methods.

On asking respondents in the survey (N = 842) why they never use spacing methods, the following factors were mentioned. A few respondents leave it all up to God:

> I am not using anything, I believe in God totally.

Other women indicated that they do not need to use spacing methods as they practice sexual abstinence:

> We follow *hasege pathya* (sexual abstinence): our birth interval is high so spacing methods are not necessary.

and others related the abstinence to religious factors:

> I do not want any more children, but I have not accepted any method. I am worshipping the Goddess Huligamma, I have devoted my life to her, so I will not get any more children.

Remarkably, of all respondents 17 per cent mentioned that they do not need to use any spacing method because they have 'natural spacing':

> I have got natural spacing.

and

> I do not become pregnant frequently.

and

> My natural interval is three years, so I did not use spacing methods.

and

> I had got natural spacing so I did not think about spacing methods: it is not necessary to use them.

The answers seem to indicate a kind of sub-fecundity, i.e. women do not conceive easily.

More than 30 per cent of the women said that they just do not know any spacing method, while another three per cent said that they do not know where to get them. Other reasons given (5 per cent) include the preference to have children as soon as possible and then undergo a sterilization.

Nine per cent of the women said they do not use spacing methods, because they do not like them or are afraid to use them. Twelve per cent of the women reported that their husbands and family members do not agree to the use of spacing methods. Another 21 per cent said that side-effects of spacing methods were a reason for non-use. We return to this in Chapter 7.

6.3 Summary and Discussion

This chapter first describes the 'fertility context' of the research area as one in which people no longer want to have as many children as possible. Respondents indicated that they desired on average only 2.7 children. The reasons are mainly economic in character: parents have to provide food, clothing and education to children, which are considered to be costly. This closely matches Caldwell's (1976 and 1982) theory on the flow of wealth: rather than children contributing to the earnings of the household, parents provide most care to the children. The quality of child rearing also plays a role: children should not only be fed, clothed and educated, but also need love and affection. Children are said to provide happiness to the family rather than contributing economically. The survival of children is still an important factor in the desired number of children, especially sons. Respondents do think that important others, especially the mother-in-law, want them to have more children than they do themselves. Again, especially the number of surviving sons is important.

Women thus definitely desire to have more sons than daughters. However, they do not desire only sons, also daughters are very much wanted. Sons are wanted for the continuation of the family line, to take care of their parents, to carry the body of the parents to the funeral place. However, daughters are wanted for help in the household but also for affection ('girls look nice in the house'). Respondents talked about the emotional attachment of daughters:

> Our sons carry our body to the funeral place, but it is our daughters who cry for us.

In addition, a few respondents indicated that although it might be that indeed sons are supposed to take care of the parents, actually daughters do so.

The majority of respondents are very well aware of the ideal duration of birth intervals. The ideal first birth interval amounts to 31 months, the ideal consecutive birth interval 36 months. Note that the actual average duration of consecutive birth intervals is 32 months. Regarding the first birth interval, about 43 per cent of women considered 24 months to be ideal, 29 per cent a duration of 36 months, whereas only 9 per cent of them preferred the first birth to occur within 23 months after marriage. With respect to the ideal interval between two consecutive births, 27 per cent of the women preferred to have a gap of 24 months, and 46 per cent a gap of 36 months. Only 1 per cent of the women thought that the next birth should occur within 23 months after the previous birth. The respondents again thought that especially their mother-in-law wanted them to have their next child within a shorter duration, i.e. after 32 months (36 months themselves).

Respondents said that the reasons for the ideal duration of the first birth interval were mainly related to their own health (especially when they marry early) and to the fact that they have to get used to their husband and his family. The reasons behind the ideal duration of consecutive birth intervals are related mostly to the health and development of the older child.

However, although women are very well aware of the ideal duration of birth intervals, quite a large proportion (40 per cent) indicated that they do not have any idea how to achieve this ideal duration. More than 3 per cent of the women stated that it is not

in their own hands, it is 'up to God' and 'in God's hands'. Almost 5 per cent of the women said they can abstain from sexual relationships. The remaining women (48 per cent) mentioned the use of a spacing method (modern or traditional), induced abortion or abortion tablets.

So, almost half of the women know that they can achieve a certain duration of birth interval by using spacing methods. Then, why is it that the reported level of ever use is only 10 per cent (see Chapter 5)? On asking women (who never used spacing methods) why they did not, 17 per cent indicated that they do not need spacing methods as they have 'natural spacing'. That is, they just do not become pregnant easily. What could this 'natural spacing' mean? As concluded in Chapter 5, important components of the birth interval are postpartum amenorrhoea, postpartum abstinence and frequency of intercourse (or sexual abstinence in general). In the following section, all three components and their probable contribution to 'natural spacing' are discussed.

On asking women what the ideal duration of postpartum amenorrhoea is, the average turns out to be 12 months. In the in-depth interviews, women mentioned that it is quite common for them to experience a duration of postpartum amenorrhoea of one or two years. The actual average duration of postpartum amenorrhoea is 9 months (see Chapter 5). On asking the women whether they knew of a link between postpartum amenorrhoea and breastfeeding, only three women (all three working in the health sector) knew about this link. The majority did not have any idea about the reason behind postpartum amenorrhoea. However, 15 per cent of the women mentioned a completely different link. That is, women lose blood during delivery, and this blood has to be restored again in the woman's body. Only when the blood is restored will menstruation start again. Some women made an extra observation: if women are not well nourished and are weak it will take more time to restore the blood and the duration of postpartum amenorrhoea thus will last longer. This is an interesting link made by the respondents themselves between nutritional status of women and the duration of postpartum amenorrhoea. The study by Ford and Kim (1993) in Bangladesh (see Chapter 2) indicates that indeed nutritional

status of the woman can determine the duration of postpartum infecundability. Among women weighing more than 44 kg, the duration of postpartum amenorrhoea was 13.6 months, among women weighing less than 38 kg 17.6 months.

When women were asked about the ideal duration of postpartum abstinence, an average of 8 months was indicated. Note that the actual average duration was 5 months (see Chapter 5). Postpartum abstinence was especially practised for the sake of the woman's health. There are many more rules regarding sexual abstinence in the research area, which are related to reproductive health events. Sexual abstinence related to abortion or sterilization is mainly practised for health reasons. Sexual abstinence during menstruation is related to ideas about pollution. However, women themselves doubt whether people really follow these rules. Estimations of the respondents themselves are that 10 per cent of the people follow the rules. Older women indicated that in former times, people followed the rules of postpartum abstinence more strictly and therefore birth intervals were longer.

In addition, rules of sexual abstinence are related to religious days and festivals, *pujas,* full and new moon days, special days in the week, etc. Abstinence is related to the polluting effect of sexual relations: one cannot approach God or provide food to God while in a polluted state. The repercussions of not following rules of sexual abstinence, as related to religion, are much more severe: family life will be affected, illnesses or disputes will occur. A common assumption is that people will obey these rules more often than the rules related to reproductive events. Respondents estimated that about 25 per cent of the people follow these religious rules of sexual abstinence.

Men further indicate that it is better not to have sex too frequently, as they lose semen and energy (*dhatu* syndrome). Also women think that too much sexual intercourse leads to weakness.

It can safely be concluded (see Chapter 5) that in the research area the duration of birth interval is mainly influenced by a relatively long duration of postpartum amenorrhoea. The long duration of postpartum amenorrhoea is due to the long duration (and frequency) of breastfeeding, and *might* also be attributed to

low nutritional status of women. As an earlier research (Hutter, 1994) indicated, more than 60 per cent of women in the reproductive ages were malnourished.

Also, different rules regarding sexual abstinence (postpartum and in general) and frequency of intercourse *might* have an influence on the duration of birth interval. However, it is not known and not measurable whether couples really adhere to the rules, and whether indeed the perception of loss of semen being equivalent to loss of energy (*dhatu*) leads to a lower frequency of intercourse. A study by Samuel (1971, cited by Singh et al., 1993) estimates, based on rules about sexual abstinence in south India, that Indian couples would refrain from sexual intercourse for between 2 and 120 days per year. By taking the rules surrounding abstinence into account, Kakar (1989: 20) concludes regarding the probability of conception in a month decreases considerably because of: 'the likelihood that most of the remaining five days are sexually safe decreases greatly'.

Finally, 17 per cent of the respondents indicate that they do not need any modern spacing method as they have natural spacing. This finding might also indicate a kind of sub-fecundity, which could be related to low nutritional status. As stated in Chapter 2, one can wonder whether the return of menses after postpartum amenorrhoea really means a return of fecundability. After return of ovulation, for example, some cycles might be irregular and sometimes anovulatory. Moreover, as Leridon (1993: 351) concludes, 'the role of the nutritional status of women is not well known'. Ford and Kim (1993) remark that the prediction of timing of return of fertility after childbirth is not an exact science and suggest heterogeneity due to other variables such as nutrition.

7

Beliefs and Perceptions about Sterilization and Spacing Methods

This chapter discusses beliefs and perceptions of women about the proximate determinant of contraceptive use. We make a distinction between beliefs and perceptions regarding sterilization and those regarding spacing methods. As indicated in Chapter 5, sterilization is very much accepted in the research area and used by 44 per cent of the respondents in the survey. On the other hand, only 10 per cent ever used a spacing method.

Section 7.1 describes the knowledge of respondents in the survey about sterilization and spacing methods, the sources of information, and whether respondents know where these are available and how much they cost. Then, following the models developed by Fishbein and Ajzen (1980) and Ajzen (1992), we examine the intentions to sterilize and practice spacing (Section 7.2.1). Also, the attitudes (Section 7.2.2), normative beliefs (Section 7.2.3) and control beliefs (Section 7.2.4) regarding sterilization and spacing methods are discussed. Section 7.2.5 provides reasons given by women as to why an intention to either sterilization or spacing behaviour was not put into practice. The aim of Section 7.3 is to get insight into the decision-making processes of those respondents who did actually use spacing methods. We focus on for example when they decided to use a spacing method, the influence of important others, the duration of use, whether health effects were experienced, etc. The information presented was collected through both survey and in-depth interviews. Details on operationalization have been discussed in Chapter 3.

7.1 KNOWLEDGE

This section examines whether respondents know about sterilization and spacing methods, the sources of information, and whether respondents know where these contraceptive methods are available and what they cost.

7.1.1 KNOWING ABOUT METHODS

We began by asking the respondent whether she knew of any method to prevent a pregnancy, and to name without prompting the methods known to her. In addition, following a list of all contraceptive methods, the respondent was asked whether she had *heard about* any of these methods (see Table 7.1).

The vast majority of respondents had knowledge about at least one family planning method: 96.7 per cent of the respondents mentioned that they knew a method. Of those who answered positively (N = 920), almost all (96 per cent) knew about sterilization.

The data achieved after probing show an even higher percentage of women who have heard about sterilization: 99 per cent. Of all women, 64 per cent have heard about Copper-T and a similar percentage about the oral pill. Only 18 per cent have heard about condoms. Half of the respondents know about

TABLE 7.1: WOMEN WHO HAVE HEARD ABOUT DIFFERENT CONTRACEPTIVE METHODS (%)

		%	N
	Yes	*No*	*NA*
Heard About:			
Sterilization	98.5	–	1.5
Copper-T	64.2	34.2	1.6
Oral pill	64.0	34.4	1.6
Vasectomy	50.8	47.5	1.7
Condom	17.7	80.8	1.6
Herbal methods	12.7	85.4	1.9
Periodic abstinence	6.0	92.1	1.9
Others	5.3	93.2	1.6

vasectomy. Thirteen per cent have heard about herbal methods, i.e. some special leaves. Only 6 per cent have heard about periodic abstinence. When this method was explained to the women, they were very eager to know more about it. Another 5 per cent of the women knew other methods, especially so-called abortion tablets which are provided by private practitioners (see Chapter 8) and injections.

Comparing the findings with the NFHS-2 of Karnataka (1998-9), knowledge of spacing methods, especially of condoms, is quite low in the research area.

More Muslim than Hindu woman have heard about the oral pill, condom and herbal method (see Table 7.2). The tribal Gouli women, living in T. Ramachandra Nagar, are less informed about all methods. Also, older women have heard more about methods than younger women. For example, while in the age group of 15-19 years 62 per cent have heard about Copper-T, the proportion of older women aged 30+ who have heard about it amounted to 74 per cent. Taking into account the contraceptive history, women who are already sterilized have heard more about spacing methods than women who have not yet been operated on and for whom knowledge would actually be more relevant. The differences between the two groups are, however, not extreme. For example, while 68 per cent of the sterilized women have heard about Copper-T, the proportion is 62 per cent for women who have not undergone the operation. For the oral pill, the proportions are 66 and 63 per cent, respectively, and for condoms 19 and 17 per cent, respectively. Differences are much more profound between illiterate and literate women. While 59 per cent of illiterate women have heard about Copper-T, for literate women this percentage is 85 per cent. Regarding the oral pill, the proportions are 61 and 78 per cent, respectively. The differences are even higher for condoms: 10 per cent for illiterate women against 46 per cent for literate women.

Women who are housewives, and especially those who are engaged in modern services and tailoring have heard more about all methods than women primarily engaged in cultivation and wage labour. Women working in modern services not only have more education (see Chapter 4) and their own income, but are usually also more exposed to information from outside.

TABLE 7.2: WOMEN WHO HAVE HEARD ABOUT DIFFERENT CONTRACEPTIVE METHODS (AFTER PROMPTING), BY VILLAGE, RELIGION, TYPE OF FAMILY (%)

	IUD	*Oral pill*	*Condom*	*Herbal*	*PerAb*	*Vasect.*	*Others*	*N*
Household Background								
Religion								
Hindu	65.2	63.0	16.9	12.4	6.3	51.1	5.4	847
Muslim	62.6	74.7	25.3	16.5	4.4	50.5	4.4	91
Christian	50.0	50.0	50.0	–	–	100.0	–	2
Gouli tribe	9.1	54.5	9.1	9.1	–	18.2	–	11
Type of Family/ Household								
Single								
Nuclear	59.6	62.8	18.6	14.2	7.6	53.3	5.7	317
Joint	63.6	62.4	17.4	11.9	6.1	45.9	5.2	327
Other	70.8	62.5	12.5	12.5	8.3	58.3	10.4	48
Co-residing								
Nuclear	72.4	70.7	15.5	12.6	3.4	55.2	4.0	174
Joint	62.7	61.3	18.7	9.3	4.0	44.0	2.7	75
Other	70.0	70.0	50.0	20.0	–	70.0	10.0	10
Individual Background								
Age group (years)								
15-19	62.3	61.0	19.2	11.6	2.1	41.8	6.2	146
20-4	60.2	63.6	14.0	10.3	4.6	46.1	4.3	349
25-9	65.9	63.7	18.1	10.9	6.9	56.8	5.4	331
30+	73.6	69.6	24.8	25.6	12.0	58.4	6.4	125
Been Operated?								
Yes	67.5	65.6	18.7	14.7	8.3	55.0	5.9	422
No	61.7	62.9	16.9	11.2	4.2	47.5	4.7	528
Literacy Level								
Illiterate	59.0	60.6	10.3	11.5	3.3	47.3	5.6	751
Literate	84.8	77.8	46.0	17.7	16.2	64.6	4.0	198

Contd.

TABLE 7.2 (Contd.)

	IUD	*Oral pill*	*Condom*	*Herbal*	*PerAb*	*Vasect.*	*Others*	*N*
Present Occupation								
Cultivation	62.1	58.1	10.1	12.3	3.5	44.1	5.7	227
Wage labour	58.2	61.4	10.8	8.8	2.3	49.7	3.6	306
Cultivation + wage labour	64.7	62.2	16.8	9.2	1.7	58.8	5.9	119
Household	68.9	69.3	25.4	16.2	10.5	50.9	7.6	228
Other	86.4	84.8	51.5	25.8	24.2	68.2	7.6	66
Exposure to:								
Radio and TV								
No	61.9	62.1	12.6	11.9	3.5	47.6	5.4	462
Yes	67.3	66.7	22.8	13.7	8.5	54.5	5.2	483
Cinema								
No	60.9	61.4	13.0	10.2	4.2	48.4	5.4	754
Yes	79.2	76.0	36.5	22.9	13.0	61.5	4.7	192
Total	64.2	64.0	17.7	12.7	6.0	50.8	5.3	
N	611	609	168	121	57	483	50	951

This can be traced to the following background variable: women who live in a household with either a radio and/or a television, have in general heard more about all methods. The differences are especially noticeable with regard to knowledge about condoms. Still, of all women who had no radio and/or television in their household, more than 60 per cent have heard about Copper-T and the oral pill. The differences in exposure become more obvious in comparing women who never visit a cinema to those who do go to the cinema. Cinema-goers have heard more about contraceptive methods.

The interviews among men (see Chapter 3) indicate that men do not know about the oral pill that can be used to avoid pregnancy. The few men who did hear about them confused the oral pill with the so-called abortion tablets. When the topic of condom came up, many men laughed about it and said they do not know anything about it. Talking about condoms is often as much a taboo as talking about sex. Just as the topic of sex is talked about through jokes, condoms are referred to through

jokes. It is strongly believed that only the promiscuous men, i.e. those who visit the town often, use condoms. 'Good' men are not supposed to talk about or use condoms. Some men have heard about condoms through the radio, some through other people talking about it. However, many have not heard of condoms. For those who have, condoms are a means to keep the gap between children and that 'the semen will not enter the female's organ if used'.

Men reported that the Auxilliary-Nurse-Midwife (ANM), whenever she visits the village, meets only the women and talks to them on all topics including family planning. There is no one who comes and talks to men about these things. Hence, the men remarked: 'how do you expect us to know more about all these things?'

7.1.2 SOURCES OF INFORMATION

Women who had heard of a family planning method were subsequently asked about their sources of information. The reported sources are classified into five broad categories, namely:

(i) interpersonal communication
(ii) health and medical personnel
(iii) non-governmental organizations (NGOs)
(iv) mass media
(v) other sources

Regarding interpersonal communication, women typically answered that they had heard about a method from acceptors, from family members, from neighbours or friends. A very typical answer was also 'village people talk about it'.

The category of health and medical personnel includes the ANM (responsible for mother-and-child healthcare in the villages), doctors and other medical personnel. The category NGOs includes especially the Family Planning Association of India (FPAI) and the India Development Service (IDS) who both work in the villages. The mass media are mainly radio and television. Other sources of information include the Anganwadi (kindergarten) worker and traditional birth attendants (TBAs).

Regarding sterilization, most respondents (73 per cent) heard

about it through interpersonal communication and another 21 per cent through health and medical personnel. Among health and medical personnel, the ANM seems to be the important source of information. NGOs and the mass media hardly play a role.

Interpersonal communication is less important as a source of information on spacing methods as compared to sterilization. Regarding Copper-T, 55 per cent of the respondents received information about the method through interpersonal com-

TABLE 7.3: WOMEN WHO HAVE HEARD ABOUT DIFFERENT CONTRACEPTIVE METHODS (AFTER PROMPTING)(%)

Source of Information	*Tub/ Lap*	*IUD*	*Oral Pill*	*Condom*	*Herbal*	*PerA*	*Vas.*	*Other*
1. *Interpersonal*	*73.3*	*55.1*	*52.4*	*39.3*	*94.1*	*56.2*	*90.1*	*76.0*
Acceptors–family	22.3	6.9	5.1	6.0	4.1	1.8	19.9	2.0
Acceptors–others	22.4	12.6	9.2	3.0	9.9	1.8	25.7	16.0
Family, husband	6.1	2.9	1.8	10.7	13.2	26.3	6.0	8.0
Neighbours/ friends	11.3	17.5	15.3	10.1	32.2	10.5	16.8	18.0
Village people	10.8	14.4	20.5	8.9	34.7	15.8	21.7	32.0
Talk in hospital	0.4	0.8	0.5	0.6	–	–	–	–
2. *Health Personnel*	*21.1*	*37.2*	*39.2*	*33.4*	*3.3*	*28.0*	*5.1*	*12.0*
ANM	17.8	32.7	34.5	26.8	0.8	17.5	3.5	6.0
Doctor	2.1	3.8	3.9	3.6	2.5	7.0	0.8	6.0
Other medical	1.2	0.7	0.8	3.0	–	3.5	0.8	–
3. *NGO*	*3.2*	*4.9*	*2.9*	*3.0*	*1.6*	*3.6*	*0.8*	–
FPAI	3.1	4.4	2.6	2.4	0.8	1.8	0.4	–
IDS	0.1	0.5	0.3	0.6	0.8	1.8	0.4	–
4. *Mass Media*	*0.5*	*1.8*	*3.6*	*22.0*	*0.8*	*5.3*	*2.5*	–
5. *Others*	*0.8*	*1.0*	*1.8*	*2.4*	–	*5.3*	*0.4*	–
Anganwadi teacher	0.6	1.0	1.6	2.4	–	5.3	0.4	–
TBA	0.2	–	0.2	–	–	–	–	–
Self	–	–	–	–	–	–	–	10.0
NA	1.0	–	–	–	–	1.8	1.0	2.0
Total N	937	611	609	168	121	57	483	50

munication, but health and medical personnel played a relatively larger role (37 per cent) compared to their role in sterilization. Again the ANM plays a major role (Table 7.3).

Regarding the oral pill, a similar pattern is observed. The NGOs, especially the FPAI, is relatively more important as a source of information on Copper-T, while the mass media are relatively more important for information on the oral pill.

Especially the higher percentage of women who have heard about condoms through the mass media is worth noting. Interpersonal communication was mentioned by 39 per cent; health personnel too was mentioned by 39 per cent.

Overall, the results signify the importance of interpersonal communication in contraceptive methods. Among health and medical personnel, the ANM plays an important role. The role of mass media is limited, but it does play a role, especially where condoms are concerned. NGOs play a minor role, as indicated by the respondents.

Taking into account the background factors, older women rely relatively more on interpersonal communication than younger women. For example, among women aged 15-19 years, 48 per cent have heard about Copper-T through interpersonal communication, compared to 63 per cent of women aged 30+. Younger women procure relatively more information about Copper-T from health and medical personnel (43 per cent against 27 per cent for older women), and about condoms from the mass media (39 per cent against 19 per cent). Also illiterate women obtain relatively more information about Copper-T, oral pill and condom through interpersonal communication. Literate women get this information relatively more through health and medical personnel, mass media, NGOs and others. The NGOs are more important as a source of information in some of the villages.

7.1.3 KNOWLEDGE ABOUT SOURCES OF SUPPLY AND COSTS

Respondents who had heard about specific methods were subsequently asked whether they knew where to obtain the methods and what the costs are. Almost all women (96 per cent) who had heard about sterilization also knew where to get it done. Of all women who have heard about Copper-T (N = 611), only

47 per cent knew where to get it, while for the oral pill this was 68 per cent. Of all women who had heard about condoms (N = 168), more than half (53 per cent) knew where to get them.

Regarding knowledge about sterilization, there is no distinction between villages, religious background, literacy level, age group, indicating how universally known sterilization is. Regarding spacing methods, the picture is different. A relatively higher percentage of Hindu women (48 per cent) know where to get Copper-T as compared to Muslim women (42 per cent). The two religious groups show no difference regarding the oral pill. More literate women and younger women know where to get

TABLE 7.4: WOMEN WHO HAVE HEARD ABOUT DIFFERENT CONTRACEPTIVE METHODS (AFTER PROMPTING), AND KNOW WHERE CONTRACEPTIVE METHODS ARE AVAILABLE (%)

	Sterilization %	*Copper-T* %	*Oral Pill* %	*Condom* %
1. *Public Sector*	*45.8*	*68.6*	*67.3*	*46.0*
Government/ municipality/ civil hospital	44.5	37.6	19.2	24.7
PHC	1.3	1.4	0.2	–
ANM	–	29.3	45.1	18.0
Anganwadi worker	–	0.3	2.8	3.3
2. *NGO*	*30.1*	*10.7*	*3.6*	2.2
FPAI	30.1	10.7	3.6	2.2
3. *Private Sector*	*1.0*	*4.4*	*15.5*	42.7
Private hospital	1.0	4.1	1.7	–
Medical shop	–	0.3	13.8	42.7
4. *Public + NGO*	*0.1*	*3.4*	*6.3*	*3.3*
Government + FPAI	0.1	3.4	6.3	3.3
5. *Public, NGO + Private*	*19.4*	*4.1*	*0.7*	*1.1*
Government + Hospital + FPAI	19.4	4.1	0.7	1.1
6. *Public + Private*	–	*0.3*	*2.7*	*3.3*
Hospital + Medical shop	–	0.3	1.2	2.2
ANM + Medical shop	–	–	1.5	1.1
7. *Other*	*3.5*	*7.9*	*3.9*	*1.1*
Any hospital/somewhere in Dharwad	3.5	7.9	3.9	1.1
Total N	903	290	412	89

Copper-T and oral pill, as compared to illiterate women and older women (30+).

Most women cited the public and NGO sectors as places where sterilization can be obtained. The public sector here consists mainly of government, civil and municipality hospitals in Dharwad, the NGO sector the FPAI (*Kutumba Yojana*). Only 1 per cent of the women mentioned a private hospital only.

The majority of women (69 per cent) named the public sector as a place to obtain a Copper-T. Again the hospitals play a dominant role, but here the ANM is also an important source. FPAI plays a minor role (11 per cent) as does the private sector (4 per cent).

The majority of women named the public sector (67 per cent) again as the place to obtain the oral pill. The ANM plays the major role (45 per cent). It is noteworthy that the role of the Anganwadi worker as a source of supply is remarkably small (3 per cent). Medical shops are another source of supply (14 per cent).

The number of women who know where condoms are available is very low (N = 89). Almost half of these women said that the public sector was a source of supply, especially the hospitals, while another 43 per cent mentioned medical shops.

If respondents knew where to get contraceptive methods, they were asked to give their estimate of the costs involved. The majority of women (69 per cent) know that sterilization is done free. Still, 22 per cent did not know the costs involved. Of the respondents, 9 per cent said that the cost was between Rs. 50 and 6,000 (private hospital). Many women said that they needed extra money for costs such as a bus ticket, extra food and medicines. Almost half of the women (48 per cent) who knew where to obtain a Copper-T and knew that they could get it free of charge. Another 46 per cent did not know the costs. More than half (53 per cent) of the women who knew where to get the oral pill and that it is available free of charge. Another 39 per cent did not know the cost, while 8 per cent mentioned amounts between Rs. 2 and 200 (medical shops). Among women who knew where to get condoms (N = 89), 40 per cent knew that they can get it free, another 52 per cent did not know, while 8 per cent gave amounts between Re. 1 and Rs. 50 (shops).

In summary, we can conclude that sterilization is well known to the respondents. Spacing methods are less well known: women have limited knowledge about the methods themselves and also about the source of supply and costs. The interviews among men indicated that they knew even less about spacing methods than women.

7.2 Models Developed by Fishbein and Ajzen (1980) and Ajzen (1991)

As explained in Chapter 2, we apply the models of Fishbein and Ajzen (1980) and Ajzen (1991) to understand and explain sterilization and spacing behaviour of women. We focus subsequently on the intention of women to use these contraceptives (Section 7.2.1); and on attitudes (Section 7.2.2), normative beliefs (Section 7.2.3) and control beliefs (Section 7.2.4) regarding sterilization and spacing methods. Section 7.2.5 presents reasons given by women about why an intention to use a method was not put into practice.

7.2.1 Intention to Use

The respondents in the survey were asked whether they had ever considered using one of the contraceptive methods, either sterilization or a spacing method. Of all respondents, 72 per cent mentioned that they did consider using a method. Note that the actual use is 44 per cent for sterilization and 10.2 per cent for spacing methods and that the percentage of women having considered using a method is thus considerably higher. Which methods did women consider using? The majority considered sterilization (65 per cent), which is a difference of more than 20 per cent points with actual use. Then, 14 per cent of the women ever considered using a spacing method (any, including periodic abstinence and other methods such as herbal methods), indicating a difference with actual use of almost 4 percentage points. The reasons why the intention was not put into practice are discussed in Section 7.2.5.

The intention to use contraceptives is influenced by attitudes, subjective norms and perceived behavioural control (Fishbein and

Ajzen, 1980; Ajzen, 1992). In the following sections we thus focus on attitudes, and normative and control beliefs.

7.2.2 Attitudes

Attitudes as defined by Fishbein and Ajzen (1980) consist of behavioural beliefs and evaluation of these beliefs. This section focuses on the behavioural beliefs defined as the expected consequences of the use of sterilization and spacing methods.

The respondents of the survey were first asked whether they thought the different contraceptive methods of sterilization, Copper-T, oral pill and condom to be acceptable, effective (i.e. can prevent a pregnancy), whether they would have health effects and whether they are convenient to use (see Table 7.5).

Almost all women find sterilization acceptable (97 per cent). Copper-T is acceptable for only 33 per cent, while almost half of

TABLE 7.5: ATTITUDES TOWARDS STERILIZATION AND SPACING METHODS

Method	*Sterilization* %	*Copper-T* %	*Oral pill* %	*Condom* %
Acceptable?				
Yes	97.1	33.2	43.8	58.9
No, against it	1.3	48.8	41.9	14.9
Don't know	0.5	14.4	10.3	24.4
Effective?				
Yes	95.7	79.5	83.3	76.8
Not at all	0.3	0.7	1.1	0.6
Don't know	0.4	18.0	11.7	19.0
Effects on Health?				
Positive effects	57.0	18.8	26.9	31.5
No effects	3.7	2.3	4.9	6.0
Negative effects	32.4	52.5	41.5	13.1
Don't know	6.5	26.4	25.9	48.8
Convenient to Use?				
Yes		36.2	60.1	52.4
Not so		13.6	13.6	5.4
Not at all		7.4	6.7	2.4
Don't know		42.9	19.0	48.8
N (heard about method)	937	611	609	168

the respondents are against the method. Oral pill is acceptable for more women (44 per cent), but still 42 per cent are against the method. Of all women who have heard of condoms (N = only 168), more than half think it is acceptable to use. The figures clearly indicate the overall acceptance of sterilization and divided attitudes about the different spacing methods.

On asking respondents whether the methods were thought to be effective, i.e. able to prevent a pregnancy, again almost all women felt that sterilization was effective (96 per cent). Most women, although to a smaller extent, also indicate that spacing methods are effective.

An important aspect is the perceived effects of use of a particular method on health. More than half (57 per cent) of the respondents thought that sterilization has positive effects on health, while 32 per cent held the opposite view. More than half of the women (53 per cent) felt that Copper-T has negative consequences for health, and for the oral pill it was 42 per cent. The percentages in the category 'don't know' are high, indicating that indeed respondents have heard about different methods but do not really know how they work and what their effects are. In the in-depth interviews, a typical comment was: 'The ANM . . . had told. But . . . I didn't know anything about it'.

Based on the literature review (Hutter, 1998), more specific questions about consequences of contraceptive methods were asked for. Almost 70 per cent of the women thought that sterilization causes weakness. Almost 30 per cent think that Copper-T would lead to bleeding (64 per cent did not know). Regarding the oral pill, 57 per cent indicated that it is 'heating' (35 per cent did not know). More than 40 per cent answered that a condom is a shame to use, 27 per cent said it is no shame and 32 per cent did not know.

The in-depth interviews subsequently revealed more clearly the perceived consequences of the different contraceptive methods.

(a) Sterilization

Table 7.6 summarizes the expected consequences of sterilization in general, as indicated by the respondents.[1] Sterilization is commonly mentioned as an operation, a tubectomy as *hoolige*

TABLE 7.6: PERCEIVED CONSEQUENCES OF STERILIZATION

Positive	– is a permanent method, to limit the number of children
	– because it is permanent, it is better than using spacing methods
	– want to get rid of this matter (of having children)
	– want to get children quickly or as soon as possible
	– feel bored with looking after more children
	– is effective
	– no more fear of pregnancy, no more fear of difficult deliveries
	– after operation women become strong
	– we can attend to our work and feel happy that we will not get any more children
	– women will be free to do any work like continuing education
	– we can do any heavy work like a man
	– we can work hard
	– we can go to the fields freely
	– we can live freely without worry
	– women become healthy if they take the right food and tonic
	– is the popular method
	– reduces our population
	– to prevent any more difficulties with pregnancy or delivery
	– is good for life's sake
Negative	– not able to work
	– difficult to lift heavy things
Leads to	– weakness
	– loss of energy
	– waist pain
	– dryness
	– leg pain
	– body ache
	– white discharge
	– death

operation (literally a stitching operation, i.e. the belly has to be 'opened' and 'closed'), a laparoscopy as a 'current operation' (referring to the electricity thought to be needed for this operation).

The effectiveness or permanency of sterilization is an important reason for women to have a sterilization. Women indicated that they preferred sterilization, to 'get rid of this matter' and 'to get

the children as quickly as possible' rather than using spacing methods. Although in general sterilization is thought to lead to weakness, some women said that they became strong after sterilization, were able to work and to 'work as a man', and in general to be free of the worries of being or becoming pregnant:

> After an operation, a woman becomes strong.

and

> If we adopt operation, we can do any heavy work like a man.

and

> After an operation, a woman will be free to do any work. . . .

However, more women report negative health effects of either a tubectomy or laparascopy:

> Now I can't work any more. . . . Pain in the legs and hands, sometimes I feel like the nerves are stuck and in the sun I have severe problems. I can't even tolerate cold. . . . I didn't have any such problem then. I was healthy earlier. After the operation all the nerves will not be normal as before. So nothing can be tolerated.

and

> I have got pain in my legs. After the operation we can't work as efficiently as earlier. I don't have pain around the waist, but I have backache and pain in my legs.

In general, weakness, a loss of energy and being dried up (*wana*) are related to sterilization in general, for both tubectomy and laparoscopy. Dryness, *wana*, literally means being dried up and indicates a general weakness (see later and Chapter 8). Some women further specified which women would face negative health effects after a sterilization:

> If a woman does not have enough blood at the time of operation, she will become weak.

The relationship between 'not enough blood in the body' and weakness is elaborated upon later (see also Chapter 8).

In addition, women say that after their sterilization operation, they cannot work hard, and certainly could not lift heavy things for a couple of months:

After I have got operated, I can't lift the pot. . . . For five months. I should not do heavy work now. I shouldn't lift pots or any other heavy things. Just light work like cleaning of the rice, etc., can be done.

Sterilization thus is reported to have negative health effects. Certain measures can be taken to ensure that women will not become weak. They are related to food intake, health check-ups, rest and abstinence from sex:

A woman should regularly take food and milk after operation.

and

During the first year after an operation a woman may need rest and she may not be in a position to work. If she can take some rest, the operation should not lead to any problem.

and

After operation we have to keep at least four months of abstinence. . . .

Given the widespread practice of sterilization—in the age group 30+ more than 80 per cent of the women were sterilized (see Chapter 5)—we can conclude that the advantages of sterilization, i.e. the permanency of the method seems to outweigh the perceived negative health effects. Women also reported the effects, often from their own experience with sterilization. Regarding spacing methods, however, the picture is different. The use of spacing methods is low and not many respondents adopted the methods. In the in-depth interviews, respondents typically talked about the effects in terms of 'hearsay', e.g.

We had *heard* that it leads to some problems.

and

They say that they can't do heavy work.

(b) Copper-T

Copper-T is called *wanki* (a traditional bracelet worn around the upper-arm) or, more affectionately, *wanki-panki*, or *ungra* (ring). Substantial negative health effects of Copper-T were cited by women in the in-depth interviews (see Table 7.7).

TABLE 7.7: CONSEQUENCES OF USING COPPER-T, AS PERCEIVED BY WOMEN

Copper-T:	
Leads to	– weakness
	– white discharge
	– tetanus
	– excess bleeding
	– septic (*nanju*), and because of septic body becomes green
	– waist pain, stomach pain
	– dryness
	– frequent stools, 'latrine problem'
	– swelling of the body; water retention in backbone
	– back pain, pain in legs and hands
	– weakness of uterus, more difficult to conceive afterwards
	– in old age, puss will form in vagina
	– may cause cancer
Other consequences	– it can kill women
	– it ruins the health of women
	– gets rusty
	– may decay
	– might go inside the stomach or to the ribs or move towards the chest
	– sticks inside and difficult to remove
	– gives trouble during intercourse: irritation for husband
	– gives trouble during intercourse: irritation or pain for woman
	– gives trouble during intercourse for husband and wife
	– moves or get displaced at time of intercourse
	– we cannot lift heavy things
	– it can be expelled while doing heavy work (making chilli powder)
	– some fat will grow next to Copper-T
	– can be used only for some time
	– difficult to remove, have to go to hospital
	– if something goes wrong, problems because difficult to remove
	– after removal, more difficult to become pregnant
	– after removal, more likelihood of abortions (miscarriages)
	– after removal, more likelihood of getting fat
	– after adoption one has to observe abstinence

Copper-T is said to lead to general health problems for women including weakness (dryness, *wana*), pain in hands and legs, pain in the stomach or waist and back pain. But more specifically Copper-T is also associated with extra bleeding, tetanus, swelling of the body or cancer. It also leads to white discharge:

> It causes white discharge. . . . Sometimes it causes pain also. . . .

Some women were so convinced about the side-effects of Copper-T that they said

> It ruins the health of women.

and

> It can kill women.

In addition, it is said that Copper-T can be septic (*nanju*), leading to infections. Others explained that Copper-T can become rusty and affects the woman's health. Another reasoning is that Copper-T can be dislocated and move up into the stomach or the chest:

> If Copper-T goes inside the body, it will be dangerous.

Some women thought that Copper-T can stick inside the body and that it is difficult to dislodge it:

> If it sticks inside, it will be difficult to remove.

Others said that Copper-T can be expelled while lifting heavy things or doing heavy work:

> If Copper-T is inserted, we cannot lift heavy things.

and

> For some women, at the time of making chilli powder, the Copper-T came outside.

Health workers later confirmed that if Copper-T is not properly inserted, it can be expelled spontaneously.

Some women stated that after insertion follow-ups are needed, which can be afforded only by rich people:

> Only rich people can afford this method; if something happens they are able to go to the hospital.

Quite a number of women indicated that Copper-T would give problems at the time of intercourse and especially create irritation and pain for the woman:

> Copper-T gets rusty (*jangu*) and will give trouble at the time of intercourse.

and

> At the time of intercourse, the woman will have trouble and get pain.

The fact that Copper-T is a temporary method is also important:

> Copper-T should get inserted and then again removed. Why to prefer this? It is an unnecessary business.

In addition, Copper-T is difficult to remove, and medical help is always needed:

> It should be removed after some time. It is difficult to go to the hospital several times to get it removed.

Also, after removal it might be more difficult to become pregnant again, and a bigger likelihood of miscarriage or developing cancer:

> The uterus becomes weak and a woman might not get another child. It may increase abortions and make us fat.

and

> The uterus becomes weak and there is a possibility of getting cancer.

(c) Oral Pill

The oral pill is called tablets (*gulige*) or by the name of the government-sponsored brand Mala-D. Like Copper-T, the oral pill is perceived to have many side-effects (see Table 7.8). Some women held strong fears of health effects:

> Women can die because of using the oral pill.

The use of the pill would lead to general weakness, extra bleeding, white discharge, dryness or weakness of the uterus. The oral pill is thought to 'dry up the body' (*wana*). This concept is reported very often, and means that the body becomes weak, that there is no strength at all (see also Chapter 8). To quote a mother-in-law:

My daughter had taken *gulige* once. But she became like a dried fish. She didn't have strength at all. But after she stopped taking them, she improved a lot.

The oral pill is considered to be heating (*ushna* or *kaavu*) and to lead to illnesses in the body related to excess heat: burning eyes, prickling sensations, skin diseases, spontaneous abortions:

I feel that the oral pill creates heat in the body. Neighbours also say this.

The concept of heating is related to the traditional Ayurveda medical system: items are classified according to the effect they have on the body, i.e. heating versus cooling, heavy versus light, dry versus moist, etc. The heating effect of the pill can be compensated by drinking cooling milk:

If a woman takes milk with tablets then it will be good, otherwise the use of pills may result in heating.

Health workers, like the ANMs and Anganwadi worker agree with the respondents that the oral pill can be heating and this effect can be compensated by the cooling effect of milk. A health worker reflects:

Nowadays every house in the village has sufficient milk. If we tell them to drink some milk after taking the tablet, they follow it. Some women can't take care. If the pill comes with severe problems, then only they stop using the tablets. . . .

One respondent related the heating qualities of the oral pill to a heating body constitution and to prolonged bleedings (see further Chapter 8):

If we take *gulige* the bleeding starts again if we are of heat constitution. Only those who don't have heat constitution can take them. . . . For women with heat constitution, it may cause bleeding again after menstruation. So I decided not to use them.

Also, it is mentioned that after the use of the oral pill it is difficult to become pregnant again. Actually, at the time of the fieldwork, the Ministry of Health and Family Welfare did not advise women who were just married to use the oral pill as it indeed might lead to infertility (see also Chapter 10).

A major disadvantage of using the oral pill is the regular daily intake. Failing in keeping this regularity might lead to unplanned pregnancies:

TABLE 7.8: PERCEIVED CONSEQUENCES OF USING THE ORAL PILL

Oral Pill:	
Leads to	– weakness – burning eyes – leg pain – swelling of the body – sepsis – tumor in the stomach – extra bleeding, more frequent periods – more pain at the time of delivery – white discharge – dryness or weakness of the uterus – difficulties in getting pregnant again, lower chances of getting pregnant again
Other consequences:	– is dangerous, can be taken for short time only – if taken for long time, woman might die – some tablets remain in the stomach and become tumor – is heating – will burn the blood – gives prickling sensation – is heating and makes woman's skin black – is heating and taken after delivery results in less breast milk for the child – is heating and might lead to miscarriages in following pregnancies – is heating but when taken together with milk or curd is no problem – is heating and thus needs to be taken with milk, which is not available in the household – makes women fat – makes women thin – makes some women fat, some women thin – makes periods regular – needs regularity of taking pills daily – if pill is forgotten for one day, not effective any more, so waste of pills – can be taken without husband or other family members knowing – is not effective, may fail – is costly, expensive to buy

It is difficult to take pills as we may sometimes forget.

Another point is that the oral pill is only for temporary use. The general idea is that two years is the maximum duration of use. If the pill is used longer it is believed to cause difficulties in conception, or women may even die:

After using pills it is difficult to deliver the next child, so I did not use it.

A positive effect of the oral pill is that it regulates menstruation:

After my second delivery I used to get my menstruation twice a month, so to maintain the regularity I used the oral pill.

Another advantage of using the oral pill is that it can be used without others noticing it:

I do not want to disclose the use of family planning to elder members of the family. That is why I am using the oral pill.

(c) Condoms

Regarding condoms, those women who knew about the method reported several side-effects, for either man or woman (Table 7.9). The most common side-effect mentioned is general weakness. The use of condoms, such as Nirodh (a government brand) too could create heat in the body of women. But more

TABLE 7.9: PERCEIVED CONSEQUENCES OF USING CONDOMS AND PERIODIC ABSTINENCE, AS PERCEIVED BY WOMEN

Condom:	
Leads to	– weakness
	– heat for women
	– weakness for men
	– effect on gents' health
Other Consequences	– shame to purchase in shop
	– not satisfactory for intercourse
	– mental dissatisfaction
	– leakage
	– not safe
	– can rupture
	– men should 'strictly follow it'

important is the shame surrounding the purchase of condoms in a shop and the dissatisfaction during intercourse:

It is a shame to purchase condoms in the shop.

and

One cannot feel satisfied during intercourse, while using condoms.

The fact that condoms are not completely safe and can leak and rupture are other perceived negative consequences of using Nirodh.

(d) Others: Periodic Abstinence

Only a few women knew about periodic abstinence. Those who knew about it mentioned that the method is good and leads to good health of both husband and wife:

By using temporary methods, a woman or man will experience some side-effects. But when we follow this traditional method we do not have any side-effects.

However, the method requires communication and cooperation between the spouses:

There should be some understanding between couples. It is better to use than all other family planning methods.

and

We cannot practise periodic abstinence regularly. It is convenient but husbands may not be ready to follow this.

and

It leads to quarrels between husband and wife.

During the fieldwork, while explaining the method, it became clear that although not many women knew about the method, there was great interest in it.

In summary, it is clear that sterilization is highly acceptable and that the positive effects (no longer pregnant, the permanency of the method) outweigh the perceived negative health effects. Women would rather choose sterilization, after having obtained the desired number of children, than use spacing methods.

Spacing methods are far less acceptable. It is not known how they work, and the (heard about) negative health effects play a very important role. In other words, the advantages of spacing methods do not outweigh the disadvantages, as with sterilization. The attitudes reported clearly do not support spacing behaviour.

Women in the in-depth interviews frequently said that spacing methods 'do not suit our body'.

Because women have to work hard, they cannot afford any side effects of a spacing method:

> We had thought of having three children one after another and then getting operated. I haven't used any spacing method. These methods don't suit us, because we have to work in the field also. We have to lift heavy containers. If we use such things, it should not result in a problem.

The ANMs whom we interviewed confirmed this observation and to an extent agreed with the respondents that spacing methods do not suit everyone. However, a general feeling among the health workers was that women in the village related their health problems to spacing methods (if used), and also to sterilization, while most of them women already had these symptoms even before they used the method. The perceived health effects of spacing methods thus were related to the general health status of women in the research area. The general health problems of women (as elaborated upon in Chapter 8) indeed were almost the same as those reported as side-effects of spacing methods and sterilization: general weakness, pain in hands and legs, pain in the back, stomach and waist and white discharge.

7.2.3 NORMATIVE BELIEFS

In order to estimate the influence of important others on contraceptive intention and behaviour of the respondents, the first question was whether the respondents discussed the methods with others (Table 7.10). Note that more than one person could be mentioned. Of all the women who had heard about sterilization (N = 937), the majority did discuss it with their husbands, 38 per cent with their mother-in-law, 51 per cent with their mother, 15 per cent with co-sister(s) and 24 per cent with neighbours or friends.

TABLE 7.10: PEOPLE WITH WHOM WOMEN (WHO HAVE HEARD ABOUT METHODS) DISCUSSED ABOUT CONTRACEPTIVE METHODS (%)

	Ever Dis-cussed	*Discussed with:* Hus-band	Mother-in-law	Father-in-law	Mother	Co-sisters	Neigh-bours	N
Sterilization	78.4	73.9	37.9	15.4	50.7	14.5	23.6	937
Copper-T	19.1	10.8	5.9	1.1	7.7	2.6	5.4	611
Oral pill	23.0	13.3	6.2	1.0	6.9	2.1	4.9	609
Condom	25.6	19.0	2.4	0	0	1.2	3.0	168

For Copper-T, oral pill and condom the picture is different. Only 19 per cent of respondents who have heard about Copper-T (N = 611) ever discussed the method with someone, 23 per cent about the oral pill, 26 per cent about condoms. Regarding Copper-T and oral pill, especially the husband, mother and mother-in-law play a major role. Where condoms are concerned, the husband was the most important discussion partner.

Women thus seem to discuss sterilization, Copper-T and oral pill predominantly with their husbands and mothers, and less with their mothers-in-law. This is remarkable, given the influence that mothers-in-law seem to have on the use of spacing methods, as indicated in Section 7.3. The percentage of respondents who discussed spacing methods with their fathers-in-law is overall low.

In addition, we asked questions (see Chapter 3) such as 'What, as you feel, does X think about you having a sterilization/using Copper-T/oral pill / condom?'

The persons included were the husband, mother-in-law, mother and neighbours or friends.

Of the women who were not yet sterilized but had heard about the method (N = 517), the majority (74 per cent) think that their husband would not agree to their having a sterilization at the time of interview (see Table 7.11). The picture is the same regarding mothers-in-law and mothers (more than 75 per cent). It is interesting that the highest percentage of agreement, according to the respondents, is to be found among neighbours or friends, i.e. 24 per cent.

Of all women who were not yet sterilized but had heard about

TABLE 7.11: RESPONDENTS WHO HAVE HEARD ABOUT CONTRACEPTIVES AND WERE NOT YET OPERATED, ACCORDING TO AGREEMENT WITH THE USE OF CONTRACEPTIVE METHODS (%)

	Agrees	*Disagrees*	*Indi-fferent*	*Don't Know*	*Some Agree*	*NA*	*N*
Sterilization							
Husband	20.7	74.3	3.3	1.2		0.6	517
Mother-in-law	12.8	76.4	6.8	3.3		0.8	399
Mother	18.0	76.2	3.2	1.7		0.9	462
Neighbours/ friends	23.8	65.4	4.8	4.3	0.2	1.6	517
Copper-T							
Husband	9.5	78.2	6.1	5.2		0.6	326
Mother-in-law	7.3	79.0	8.5	4.4		0.8	248
Mother	6.6	84.7	6.3	1.7		0.7	287
Neighbours/ friends	11.7	72.1	8.9	4.9	0.9	0.6	326
Oral Pill							
Husband	13.3	74.4	9.0	2.7		0.6	332
Mother-in-law	7.8	74.5	9.8	7.1		0.8	255
Mother	10.9	78.9	7.5	2.0		0.7	294
Neighbours/ friends	15.4	67.8	10.2	5.7	0.3	0.6	332
Condom							
Husband	31.5	41.6	6.7	18.0		2.2	89
Mother-in-law	7.0	46.5	21.1	23.9		1.4	71
Mother	8.2	42.5	20.5	27.4		1.4	73
Neighbours/ friends	14.6	36.0	12.4	30.3	1.1	5.6	89

Copper-T (N = 326), 79 per cent think that their husbands will not agree to their using Copper-T. Similar, or even higher percentages are reported for the mothers-in-law and mothers. A similar pattern is discerned for the use of oral pill, although the percentages of respondents who think their husband, mother-in-law, mother and neighbours or friends would agree to their using the oral pill, are a bit higher than for Copper-T.

Of all respondents who were not yet sterilized but had heard about condoms (N = 89), more than 30 per cent think that their husbands would agree to use condoms while 42 per cent think that they would not agree.

According to the data about all contraceptive methods, the majority of the respondents think that the people in their immediate environment would not agree to their use of a method.

In conclusion, the normative beliefs are not very supportive of the use of spacing methods. In the in-depth interviews several women said that they were not allowed by either mother-in-law, elders or husband, to use spacing methods:

> I didn't get my menstruation for one year. Then the ANM told me to take those Mala-D tablets, to postpone pregnancy. But it was not accepted in our house. So I didn't take them. It is said that the tablets cause heat in the body. So they didn't agree to it. I didn't even think of it. I asked my mother-in-law about the tablets when the ANM told me. But she said not to take them. So I dropped the idea.

and

> My husband didn't allow me to take pills. I had heard people talk about pills. But he did not allow me to take them. Instead he told me to get operated later on and I got operated. Even if I wanted, my husband didn't allow me, because he thinks that it would lead to some problem in future. If it doesn't lead to any problem it is good. But we don't know the side-effects. In villages they don't remember the dates and all that. If by mistake we take pills in third or fourth month, that leads to problems. So, I was not allowed.

7.2.4 CONTROL BELIEFS

Perceived behavioural control, or more particularly the control beliefs are operationalized (see Chapter 3) by two questions: whether women think it is easy to see providers of contraceptives and get the contraceptives. And, whether women think they can afford to pay the costs of contraceptives. The questions could only be posed to those respondents who knew where to get the different methods, and those who knew the costs of the different methods, respectively (see Section 7.2.1).

Of the respondents who knew where sterilization can be obtained (N = 903), the majority (69 per cent) found it easy to go to the hospital or clinic for a sterilization, while 20 per cent found it not so easy, and only 9 per cent thought that it was very difficult (see Table 7.12). Of all respondents who knew where to get Copper-T (N = 290), almost 70 per cent thought that it was easy

TABLE 7.12 : WOMEN WHO KNEW WHERE CONTRACEPTIVES WERE AVAILABLE AND THEIR PERCEPTION OF THE ACCESSIBILITY OF CONTRACEPTIVES (%)

Easy to go and get?	*Easy*	*Not So Easy*	*Very Difficult*	*Don't know*	*NA*	*N*
Method						
Sterilization	68.9	20.4	8.7	1.9	0.1	903
Copper-T	69.3	14.5	3.8	11.4	1.0	290
Oral pill	81.3	9.2	3.2	3.6	2.7	412
Condom	74.2	9.0	4.5	9.0	3.4	89

to go to the providers and get a Copper-T inserted, 4 per cent found it difficult and 11 per cent just did not know. Of all respondents who knew where to obtain the oral pill (N = 412), more than 80 per cent thought that it was easy to go and get the pill, and only 3 per cent said that it was difficult. Of all respondents who knew where to get condoms (N = 89), 74 per cent said it was easy for them to obtain condoms.

We can conclude that unlike attitudes and normative beliefs, control beliefs are supportive of the use of spacing methods: respondents who knew about the methods and knew where to get them, do not find it difficult to go to the providers and ask for them. Note that all methods are provided free by the ANM and government services.

Of all respondents who knew the costs of a sterilization (N = 706), the majority (77 per cent) also found it easy to pay these costs, while 10 per cent found it very difficult (Table 7.13). Of all respondents who knew the costs of Copper-T (N = 157),

TABLE 7.13: WOMEN WHO KNEW ABOUT THE COSTS OF CONTRACEPTIVES, AND THEIR PERCEPTION OF EASE TO PAY THESE COSTS (%)

Easy to Pay?	*Easy*	*Not so Easy*	*Very Difficult*	*Don't Know*	*NA*	*N*
Method						
Sterilization	76.5	12.2	9.8	0.7	0.8	706
Copper-T	84.7	5.7	2.5	1.9	5.1	157
Oral pill	91.5	6.5	1.2	–	0.8	248
Condom	90.5	7.1	–	–	2.4	42

85 per cent thought it is easy to pay the costs, and only 3 per cent found it difficult. Of all respondents who knew the costs of oral pill (N = 248), more than 90 per cent said that it was easy to pay for; only 1 per cent found it difficult. The same proportion applied to condoms (N = 42 only). In summary, the costs of spacing methods do not pose a real obstacle to usage.

7.2.5 FROM INTENTION TO BEHAVIOUR

Section 7.2.1 showed that quite a number of women intended to use a contraceptive method but did not actually use them. This refers to sterilization as well as spacing methods. For sterilization, the difference between intention to use and actual use is higher (65 per cent versus 44 per cent) than for spacing methods (14 per cent versus 10 per cent).

What are the reasons, as reported by women, for intending to use a method but not actually using it? It should be noted here that sterilizations are usually conducted immediately after delivery. If a woman is not sterilized after a delivery, commonly she will wait until the next child is born. Having a sterilization some time after delivery does not seem to be an option.

A major reason why respondents do not have a sterilization after a delivery, although they intended to have it, is the sex of the child born. If the child is not a boy, parents might decide—depending on the sex composition of the family—to delay a sterilization until the following delivery:

> I wanted to go for an operation after the last delivery. As it was also a female baby, I postponed it to the next delivery. I want to have a male child.

The same can happen, but less frequently, when a daughter is wanted:

> I wanted to adopt operation after the second child, if it was a girl. But it was a boy, so I was not operated after the second child.

It is not necessarily the respondent herself who decides to postpone the sterilization. The influence of mothers-in-law, husbands and mothers is evident:

> I wanted to adopt operation after the second living child, but my mother-in-law (*atte*) did not allow me, because she wants one more male child.

and

I wanted to go for an operation after the second child, but my husband disagreed as he wanted to have a female child. So I did not go.

and

I was ready to go for an operation after the last delivery. My mother opposed and insisted on one more boy child.

Not only are women dependent on others, but husbands are also dependent (although to a lesser extent than women) on elders. One of the male respondents indicated:

I wanted to get the operation done to my wife after the first child. I also gave that in writing. Elders in the neighbourhood and my in-laws opposed and asked me to get one more son. Elders did not give me consent. . . .

and

I wanted to get tubectomy operation done to my wife after the birth of the second child. . . . My wife's name was also registered with the government hospital nurse. After 8 days, the nurse came with the jeep to take my wife for the operation. Then, I went to call my father-in-law and mother-in-law. The father-in-law came and vehemently said 'Who told you to take her for operation? Are we not there for you? You did not tell a single word to us. I will not send her for an operation. I will pay your expenditure.' My father and mother also told me that since you have only one son, you can get her stomach burnt (laproscopy) after one more child whether it is male or female.

It is remarkable that almost none of the women mentioned that others wanted them to have a sterilization when they themselves did not want to.

Another reason not to undergo a sterilization as intended is related to the health and survival of the children:

I wanted to have an operation after the second child. But then I lost this child when it was three days old. So I dropped the idea of an operation after the second child. Now I want two more children.

and

After my second delivery I thought of having an operation. But after two years I lost my child. So after one more child I am going for an operation.

Related to this, some young respondents mentioned that medical

personnel did not want them to undergo sterilization because the children were still young, and might not survive. In some instances, women themselves were considered to be too young:

> I have sufficient children, and I wanted to have an operation. As I am still young, the doctor is not ready to operate.

and

> I wanted to have only two children. But my first son was too young at the time of my second delivery; he could not even walk. So, the doctor was not ready to operate on me.

Quite often women are unable to undergo a sterilization, as indicated by health personnel, because of severe anaemia. Women are then advised to first improve their health.

The interviews illustrate that women start thinking about sterilization quite early in their reproductive career: respondents talk about an operation

> 'after two more children'
> 'after one boy'
> 'after the next delivery', etc.

The interviews also indicate that women decide, together with their husbands and family members, in a 'strategic', rational way, taking into account, for example, the possibilities of survival of their children and the need to have at least one son.

With regard to spacing methods, there are fewer examples of why an intention to use spacing methods is not translated into actual spacing behaviour. The difference in percentages between actual use (10 per cent) and intended use (14 per cent) is also lower than for sterilization. One factor is that spacing methods often can be used—according to medical personnel and personnel of the Family Welfare Department—after the period of postpartum amenorrhoea, i.e. when menstruation resumes. Women who thought about using spacing methods indicated that they started thinking about using a method only at that time. Some respondents turned out to be pregnant already before they could start using the spacing methods:

> I was still not having my periods, so I did not think about using oral pill or Copper-T.

and

> After delivery, I did not get my periods yet. After getting my periods back, I want to use a temporary method but I did not yet think about that.

7.3 Decision-making Processes: Use of Spacing Methods

After having discussed so many aspects and reasons why women do *not* use spacing methods, who are the women who ever used spacing methods? In this section a number of case studies are presented in order to get more insight into the decision-making processes of women who actually used spacing methods. The focus is on questions such as: *when* they decided to use a spacing method; what was the *duration* of use; how the *decision* to use spacing methods was *made*; what was the *influence* of important others; whether *health effects* were experienced, etc. The case studies are presented first, followed by a summary.

Case Study 1

The in-depth interviews indicated that few women were able to decide for themselves the use of a spacing method. C, who seems to be completely in control of her life, planning all her pregnancies, is an exception. At the time of the interview, C was 26 years old and part of the group of Scheduled Tribes. She used the oral pill after the birth of her first child (daughter) and second child (son).

Timing and Duration of Use

C started to use the oral pill while she stayed in her mother's place at the time of delivery of her first child:

> I used to take them after delivery, because I got my periods 20 days after delivery. I started to take the oral pill when I started to live together with my husband. . . . Because I started to menstruate very soon after delivery.

She used the pill for about two years:

> When I wanted to have a child, I stopped taking them.

Influence of Other People

She got to know about the pill, around that time, through her sister, who was working in an Anganwadi school:

After the delivery, I told my sister (in *tavaru mane*) that I had started to get my periods and asked her what should I do. She was working in a school, so she knew about the pill. She told me to ask the ANM about it.

She herself asked the ANM about the pill:

I asked her myself. I told her that I had heard about such pills and I wantded to take them. She gave them to me.

The ANM brought her the package of oral pills every month:

I didn't ask anybody and I didn't tell anybody. I had asked only my sister. The ANM came regularly. Once we registered the name with her, she used to give the tablets monthly. We had to meet her every month after my menstruation.

C said that both her husband and mother-in-law did not know that she was using oral pills (*gulige*). Only very recently, her husband and mother had got to know about it:

I have told them about it now, just two days back. I had gone to a neighbour's house. She had conceived very soon after marriage. So everybody was teasing her. Then somebody asked me. I said that I was taking the oral pill. They didn't say anything. . . . My husband knows. My mother-in-law (*atte*) doesn't know. Now my mother knows. . . . She said that it was good . . . then . . . she would have said 'no', because she is a village woman and of old ideas.

Why was she so determined to use the oral pill?

Not to get children very soon one after another. I didn't want to get a child every year. If I got one who would look after us? With small children it is very difficult.

Difficult to Take Oral Pill?

In reply to the question about whether it is difficult to use the oral pill (taking a tablet every day) while living with a family who does not know that she is taking them, C answered:

I used to take the oral pill daily after the dinner.

And to the question whether people did not see her using them, she replied:

In our house nobody does like that. In some houses the others will ask as to what this is and that, etc. But in our house it is not so.

CASE STUDY 2

The second respondent is 17 years old and has one son. She used the oral pill after her husband advised her to do so.

Timing and Duration of Use

She started to use the oral pill:

After the birth of the boy. He was eight or nine months old.

Selecting a Method

For the question why she used oral pill, the respondent made a comparison between the oral pill and other spacing methods:

It is said that with Copper-T there are more problems. . . . It is said that the body dries up (*wana*).

Wana literally means dry, but here it means weakness, not having any strength (refer to preceding and Chapter 8).

Influence of Other People

The decision to use the oral pill was taken on her own, after she had been advised by her husband. The ANM gave her the tablets.

My husband told. The ANM comes weekly once, she gives the tablets.

At that moment, her mother-in-law and others did not know that she used the oral pill. Like in the first case study, later the family-in-law admitted that it was a good thing to do:

. . . We decided ourselves. Now, they say it is a good thing that we did so.

CASE STUDY 3

Another respondent, who was 18 years old at time of interview, got her first daughter within the first year of marriage. Her second daughter was born within 1.5 years. S used Copper-T after her second child. Her mother-in-law told her to do so and she 'obeyed'.

Timing and Duration of Use

I had a Copper-T (*wanki*) inserted and used it for a year and a half. But I got it removed one month back.

Influence of Other People

The mother-in-law played an important role:

My mother-in-law told me to use it. . . . If we give birth every year to a child, then it will become a problem to manage everything. There is only one earning person in the family. If there are more children it is difficult to feed them. Moreover we don't have any property. So it will be better if there is a little gap.

Her mother-in-law got the information from the ANM and the Anganwadi worker:

The ANM had told about it. She comes to the Anganwadi worker's house. She had told my mother-in law about oral pill and Copper-T.

S did not dare tell her husband that she was using Copper-T:

No, he didn't know about it . . . she (mother-in-law) had told me to tell to my husband. But I felt shy and didn't tell him.

Later, when she told him:

He didn't say anything.

Later in the interview S added that she was afraid that he would not agree:

. . . If I told him earlier there was a chance for him to say no.

The mother-in-law seems not really to be an advisor but someone whose orders have to be obeyed:

We obey the elders. When she told me to do so, I accepted it. But later when the problems started I told her only. She told me to get it removed.

Selection of Method

On asking whether she considered using another spacing method, e.g. the oral pill, S replied

It is said that the body dries up due to the oral pill . . . but it is also said that due to Copper-T the body dries up.

She actually feels that no method is really good.

Health Effects?

S experienced quite a number of side-effects. She attributes the problems to Copper-T because when she got it removed her problems disappeared:

Pain in hands and legs, backache, stomach pain, etc. . . . now that I have got it removed at present I don't have any problems. After its removal, if I become pregnant again, we have decided to have the baby and then get operated.

Discontinuation

S got her Copper-T removed only recently. She did not think about another method to use:

I didn't ask about the other methods. My mother-in-low told me to continue with the Copper-T. But I could not, because I had problems with it.

Did the ANM remove it?

Yes.

Case Study 4

The respondent related in detail about the decision-making process in using spacing methods, during several birth intervals. She used the oral pill for the first time after the birth of her first daughter.

First Time Use: Timing and Duration

I have taken tablets and also injections. . . . I took them for one year after the first delivery.

She decided to use the pills the moment her menstruation started again:

. . . I told her (ANM) that I got the menstruation back after six months. So she told me to use the tables to postpone pregnancy. I told my grandmother what the ANM had said. She agreed to it.

A is married to her *sodermaava* (mother's brother) and as a consequence her mother-in-law is her grandmother.

She discontinued the tablets after one year:

Then the elders in our house said that the first child had grown. So they felt even if I conceived again, it would not be a problem. So they told me to stop the tablets. . . . My grandmother told me to stop them. She said it may lead to problems if I took them for a longer period.

Influence of People

When asked who told her about the pill, A answered:

The ANM. . . . She had told me to take these tablets. Otherwise I would conceive and bear children very early. She told me that I can stop using the tablets later. I agreed and took them.

Before starting to use the oral pill, A asked permission from her mother-in-law:

I had told her (ANM) that I would have to ask my grandmother. . . . My grandmother knew about it. Before using the tablets, I had also told her.

On asking what she would have done if her mother-in-law had not agreed:

I would not have taken those tablets. We can't disobey our elders.

The ANM brought the packages to her home every month:

She brought them (oral pill) along with her. Even if I was not at home, she would give them to my grandmother (actually her mother-in-law). Anyway she knew about it. If the elders in our house know about it, they can give

the tablets to them. If they don't know about it, then we have to get them secretly.

Her husband did not know, and still does not, that she used the oral pill.

On asking A how her *atte* knew about the oral pill and agreed to let her use them A said:

The ANM is known to our family. My *sannavva* was working in the Anganwadi. She knew the ANM better. The ANM came to our house often. So she was known to our family, like her (pointing at the researcher) . . . for many years socially recognised people have visited this house. That is the main reason why my grandmother agreed to the tablets.

Health Effects?

In contrast with the previous respondent, A did not have any difficulties while using oral pill:

No. I didn't have any problem.

Difficult to Take?

On asking whether A found it difficult to take the pill on a regular basis, a reason expressed by respondents who never used oral pill, she said that she did not have any problem:

No. I took them regularly. There was some mark on the pack and I had to take them according to the given direction. There was some number and I had to start them from there.

On asking where she kept the pill, as her husband did not know about her use:

I kept them in another room. . . . After finishing all the kitchen work, I used to take the tablets and then go to our room. . . . He didn't see them. Even if he had seen them, he would not ask anything about it.

Reasons for Using

A is very well aware of the negative health effects of having children too soon after each other:

If we don't, we will be the sufferers. If we conceive again, when the first child is very small, we can't take care of it and also we can't work efficiently. We can't go to work also if we conceive when the previous child is very young. If there is some gap between the children, that child can eat by itself and we also can look after our work. Then the pregnancy will not be a burden. So to be on the safe side, we have to take those tablets. So I took those tablets.

Second Time Use: Timing and Duration

After the birth of her second daughter too, A took the oral pill. However, she could use the oral pill then for only six months, because the ANM allegedly did not provide the tablets on a longer basis. A relates it to the policy of the government, represented at the local level by the ANM, which states that oral pill should not be provided to women who already have two children:

They told me that they didn't have permission to give tablets to those having two children. . . . I felt what can I do if she doesn't give the tablets. We will leave it to fate. If I conceive again, I cannot not help it and if the menstruation continues it is better.

On our question whether she did not ask the ANM about it, the answer was:

No. Because if she gets them from the government she would give us the tablets. Otherwise how can she give us the tablets?

A could have thought about using another spacing method, after six months, but she did not want to:

She (ANM) had told about *wanki*. But I didn't accept it. . . . I had the feeling that it would create problems later. I had heard from a woman that she got some problem after using wanki. . . . She said that the *wanki* had rusted inside and as a result there was some problem. After that she was not well. Since hearing that I was not ready to use it.

Third Time Use: Timing and Duration

After the third delivery, a son, A did not take tablets as they were not provided to women with three children:

They said that they would not give tablets after every delivery. They said that only after the first two deliveries we give you the tablets. After the third delivery they didn't give the tablets. They told that after 2-3 children, it is better to get operated or to use the loop. The tablets are not good after three deliveries, they said. Government doesn't allow that.

A considered sterilization but her family liked her to have one more son:

Actually I wanted to get operated after my son. But my grandmother and *doddavva* (mother's elder sister) didn't agree. They didn't want me to have only one son. I conceived again when the boy was 1½ years old and I delivered another girl when he was 2 years 3 months old. After that I firmly decided and got operated. . . .

The elders told her to wait again for one more son:

They told. But I didn't listen to them. If I continued to get one girl after another. . . . What could I do? So I told them that according to my fate I have only one son and I have had enough children now. So I wanted to get operated.

A thus ended up with four children: three daughters and one son.

Convincing Other Women in the Reproductive Age

We asked A whether she, having lots of experience in using the oral pill and—as she herself stated—and belonging to a socially recognized family, provided any information about *gulige* to other women in the village. It turns out, as in later case studies as well, that women in the reproductive ages do not tell other women in their own age group about spacing methods:

No. I don't tell other women, because I will not think like you and you will not think like me. Moreover the elders in the house will be thinking differently, even if we agree to it. So, we use it ourselves. We don't tell others. The elders will ask who gave it, why did they give, etc. They will scold me. We don't like that.

On asking whether she told anyone in her family then, A reveals that she certainly cannot tell her sister who recently got married:

I haven't told anybody. Recently my younger sister got married and went to her husband's house. So at that time I told her how she should behave in her

husband's house. We tell others only things which can be told. We don't talk about such things.

CASE STUDY 5

This case study again illustrates the important role played by the mother-on-law and the ANM. The respondent D, Muslim by religion, said that she did not use any spacing method in the period that her first three children were born. Now, having one son and three daughters, she decided to use the oral pill.

Reason for Not Using, Influence Other People

D's first reason was that she did not have knowledge about them:

Then (earlier) we didn't know. If we knew about it, we could have done something. Now the ANMs give more information about it . . . then the information was less.

However, she said that her mother-in-law (*atte*), with whom she lived at that time, had a negative attitude towards the ANM:

Whenever the ANM came to our house, my *atte* used to tell her that we want more children as we have land and sent her away and we did not go out at all.

D, only got access to the ANM after she moved to a separate house, away from her mother-in-law:

My *atte* used to sit at the front door and used to send the ANM away by telling her that nobody was at home. . . .

It was the ANM who gave D the oral pill:

The ANM gave Mala-D tablets.

Her sister told her about the tablets during her stay in her mother's place after delivery:

My sister told me to take them as she was also using them. I had gone for delivery to my mother's house and she had also come there. She told me that it would be better to use the tablets because all my children were very young.

Her husband was informed only later, although he seemed to know that she was using the pill:

> He knew. But didn't say anything to me. I didn't ask him before using them.

Timing and Duration

D was convinced about the oral pill and told the ANM that she wanted to use them. The ANM, however, told her to wait until her menstruation started again after delivery:

> The ANM told me to wait till I got back my menstruation. She told me to go to her after I get my menstruation for the tablets . . . (I started) 8-9 months after the delivery.

She used the oral pill for two years.

Problems Faced

D did not face any problems in using the oral pill, on the contrary:

> . . . . Actually I felt good by using them.

On remarking that some women say that it causes heat, D said:

> Yes. Many women say that. But I had decided to use them, and ignore its side-effects. But I benefited by using them.

This is an interesting remark, which seems to indicate that once the benefit of not becoming pregnant (or being free of the fear of becoming pregnant) is clear, possible side-effects are 'ignored' or not felt.

Discontinuation

However, she did experience some side-effects and she discontinued the oral pill because of the heating effects:

> The effect of heat was too much. So I had to stop. . . . Due to heat I did not feel well. I used to feel heat inside the abdomen also.

The concept of heat is related to the traditional medical system of Ayurveda and is described in detail in Chapter 8.

CASE STUDY 6

The present respondent Y used the oral pill and said that she had difficulties conceiving again.

Timing and Duration

Nine months after her delivery, due to some problems Y had to leave—her daughter in her brother's place. She started to use the oral pill then.

After leaving that child there, I was afraid of conceiving again. Then it would be problematic. So I took Mala-D tablets for one year. Two years after the delivery I got my periods back. As I was afraid of conceiving again I took Mala-D tablets for one year. After that I have not conceived. I took them only for one year. . . . I stopped the tablets thinking that it would be proper if I conceived again but it would be alright if I didn't conceive either.

Health Effects

When asked whether she had any problems using the pill:

No. I took on my own decision and I stopped them on my own. I took them for one year.

When we asked her about the common perception that the oral pill is heating, she replied that she always has had a heating body constitution and that she cannot blame the tablets for those heating effects (unlike the former respondent):

But my constitution is of heat since many years. The skin of my heels crack and sometimes ulcers appear in mouth. But my constitution is like that only. After menarche I didn't get periods regularly every month. Once in two or three or four months. At the maximum I menstruate 4-5 times in a year.

On asking whether her inability to conceive could be related to the use of the oral pill, which was the opinion of the other respondent, she disagreed. She did not blame the tablets, nor the ANM, as she has always had this constitution:

Some women say that. What I say is that since menarche I have such a problem. I took the tablets for my benefit. How can I blame the ANM for

that? I know that I have this problem since menarche. Now I don't feel that I must get children. Whether I get children now or not doesn't matter.

It is quite interesting that this respondent does not relate her health problems to the use of the oral pill, while—as seen before—so many women do relate spacing methods with general health problems such as weakness and infertility.

Influence of other People

Y did tell her husband that she was using the oral pill:

I had told him about it before I started them. Both my brother and my husband knew about it. I had consulted him (husband) before taking tablets. He agreed to it. The ANM told me how to take those tablets.

She said that she and her husband are the only earners in the house. That is why she wanted to postpone another pregnancy, by taking oral pills:

If women have others at home to take care of children, they don't think of using the oral pill to postpone pregnancy. Some parents will be ready to take the responsibility of even third or fourth deliveries. In such a case women need not think about postponing pregnancy. I have a sister. She has a job. So she can take leave at the most only for one month. For one month after the delivery she can take care of us, after that we have to come to the husband's house and we have to carry on all the domestic responsibilities in *hasi mai* only.

Y's mother-in-law was not informed about her using the oral pill. Now that Y, is not able to conceive, her mother-in-law blames the tablets, and thus Y, for having taken them:

She came to know about it very recently, when for a long period I didn't conceive. Just as I am telling you now about it, some time ago I told one of my neighbours, and the news spread from one woman to another. Thus my mother-in-law came to know about it and she says that only because of those tablets I can't conceive. . . . They scold me because I took the tablets.

CASE STUDY 7

Quite another reason to use spacing methods is provided by K, the next respondent, aged 29 and with one daughter and one son.

She used copper-T after the births of her children. Instead of undergoing a sterilization immediately after the second child, she was advised to wait for some years and to use a 'spacing' method. Once it was more or less certain that her two children would survive, she would go for sterilization.

Timing and Duration

The respondent used Copper-T after her second child, a daughter, was born:

> I used Copper-T. I got it removed after three years and got operated. My son was young and I had got the daughter already.

She was still in her mother's place after her delivery:

> The ANM told me to use something. I was still in my *tavaru maṅe* and she came there only and inserted it.

Operation Postponement

Knowing the general preference for a sterilization immediately after a delivery (so that the care provided to a wet mother can be combined with the care needed after sterilization), we asked whether a sterilization some years after delivery is not considered to be more difficult?

> I preferred to get operated after my children grew a little. I have undergone the current operation.That didn't cause much problem. If we undergo tubectomy, then it has to be done soon after delivery. But for laparoscopy it is not so. Therefore I preferred this. But I don't have any problem and it has also not failed. Among women who are thin, it doesn't fail. But among women who are fat it fails often. But we don't have any problem.

Influence other People?

Medical professionals, especially the ANM and a doctor in the hospital advised her to use a spacing method and postpone sterilization:

> . . . She (ANM) told me to use it to delay the conception and to get operated later. . . . One month after delivery I got it inserted. I had gone to the hospital

to get operated, but the doctor told me that it was better to wait until the son was 5 years old. Till then, he would not operate. He suggested to use *wanki*. All both the children had grown a little. Then after three years I went to the hospital . . . and got it removed.

K herself decided to have the Copper-T inserted. She did not ask permission from her husband, but he agreed:

He agreed to it because otherwise we would have children too frequently. I didn't ask anybody. I decided myself to get it inserted, to avoid getting children one after another.

K's mother did not agree, and her mother-in-law silently accepted it:

At that time my father was there; my mother was not there. After she came back she came to know about it and started to blamee. . . . My mother-in-law didn't say anything. She asked me once why I was using it. But I told her it is not good if I get children very often. She agreed.

Health Effects

K did not face any health problems, although her mother told her about side-effects:

She told me that the blood will get burnt by using such things. Some people get adjusted to it and some not.

On asking K whether this strategy (i.e. having children and using spacing methods before a sterilization is conducted) is adopted by more women in the villages, she answered positive and elaborated:

Yes. There are many women who go for operation after some time, because there is uncertainty about the life of the children. Those who conceive frequently or those who have 4-5 children may not wait till their children grow a little. But women like me who have only 1-2 children wait for three years before going for operation. I now have one son and one daughter.

Case Study 8

Sometimes the strategy adopted by a respondent, like M, aged 21, does not work out. M wanted to undergo sterilization after

one daughter and one son were born. However, both medical professionals and her family made it impossible for her to follow her own strategy. The case study illustrates the strong social pressure put upon young women in the reproductive age.

Timing and Duration

M used Copper-T after her second child, a daughter, was born, for a period of three years. She wanted to have a sterilization after the delivery of her daughter but the ANM convinced her not to have it immediately:

> Both of them (the children) were very young. So the ANM advised me not get operated. So I dropped the idea then. Some time in between I again wanted to go for the operation. The ANM told me that the operation can be done later, and that it was better to use Copper-T. I agreed and got it inserted for three years. . . . I started to use it five months after delivery. During the third month my periods started again.

Influence of other People

M's husband also thought about sterilization after the delivery of the second child:

> He had also told me to get operated. But because the children were young then, it was not possible. The family members also didn't agree to it.

M got her Copper-T inserted in a family planning clinic in Dharwad where the medical professionals—like the ANM earlier—also told her that she could not have a sterilization:

> There the doctors themselves told that. My eldest daughter was one year old when the second child was born. But because the children were very young, they were not ready. If my children were not so young. I would have not listened to anybody. I would have got operated.

She regrets that she could not make the decision to have an operation:

> I didn't want to listen to others.

Later during the interview, she said that it was actually her mother-in-law, TBA in the village, who told her to use Copper-T.

Health Effects of Copper-T

M had health problems related to the use of Copper-T:

> I had problems of waist pain and white discharge. So I got it removed.

Discontinuation

M used the Copper-T for three years. She herself wanted to have it removed earlier. But when she complained about the health effects and wanted it to be removed, the ANM refused to take it out:

> She had told me that it can be taken out even before. . . . I told her many times to take it out. But she kept on saying something about completing three years. I wanted to get it out because of the waist pain. For many days she didn't come here. . . .

M thus visited another health service clinic to get it removed:

> Not every woman adjusts to Copper-T. It was the same for me. So I wanted to get it removed, but they didn't remove it. They told me that it would be waste of government money and that my problem was not severe. Only six months had passed since I had got it inserted. But later when I started to become very thin, my *akka* (older sister) told me to get it removed in a private nursing home. We went there to get it removed. There the doctor told me that it didn't suit me.

After Discontinuation, Sterilization?

After three years of use, M's Copper-T was removed. Then she wanted to go for a sterilization. However, her in-laws did not agree and told her that it is good to conduct a sterilization only soon after a delivery. As indicated before, most sterilizations are conducted soon after delivery so that the care to be provided after a sterilization can be combined with the care to be provided to a nursing mother. M did not go for a sterilization then and was pregnant at the time of the interview:

> After the delivery I wanted to get operated, but instead started using Copper-T. Actually I didn't want to use Copper-T; I wanted to get operated. But the ANM didn't agree to it. The elders in the house too didn't agree and it was told that the operation will be good only after delivery. So, I kept quiet. But now I have conceived again.

I conceived five to six months after I got it removed . . . our family members said to get operated after one more child. . . . I am four months pregnant now.

Both the age of her two children, a boy and a girl, and the health status of the girl played a role in shaping the opinion of the elders that M should not to be operated:

If the children were not so young then, I would have got operated definitely. But my children were very young. The daughter was not keeping well, because I had delivered another child a year after she was born. I could not feed her properly. She was very ill.

Case Study 9

An exceptional case is an educated respondent who used condoms after the birth of two children: one son who died when he was a couple of months old and one girl.

Timing and Duration

M started using condoms 1.5 years after the birth of her second child. She was in postpartum amenorrhoea for one year, which is considered to be quite normal:

I . . . got my menstruation only one year after delivery and for my sisters it was 2-3 years.

M said that she was worried about becoming pregnant again:

After the first delivery I had conceived soon. So I worried that if I get my menstruation again after one year, l would conceive again.

Her husband used condoms for one year.

Influence of Other People

It was the ANM who told M to have a gap between the children and who suggested condoms and also provided them:

The ANM told me to have a gap of three years between two children. Otherwise I would have got one more child now. After her advice we started to use Nirodh.

After the ANM advised her, M herself told her husband about using condoms:

He agreed readily to it, because there are only 2 of us at home. There is nobody to take care of us. If we get children one after other it creates problem either for him or me. This was the first time that we used them.

What did her Husband Say?

He didn't say anything. I told him that the ANM had advised me to use it in order to postpone the pregnancy, because our girl was very young. It would be problematic if we got more children. He agreed. He is also educated and understands the problem. In villages the uneducated people are not ready to use them. They feel it better to get 3-4 children.

M then added an important point, i.e. that they only started to use the condoms after beginning to live on their own:

We had separated then. We started to use it after we came to this house. Earlier we had to go the fields for work sometimes. Such things would not be allowed there.

M's family does not know that they are using condoms:

Now . . . they say that I haven't conceived for a long period. My father and my mother-in-law often mention it. I told them that I get children whenever God gives. I didn't tell them that we were using Nirodh.

Difficult to Dispose of?

One of the reasons for the low use of condoms, as suggested in other interviews, would be that they are difficult to dispose of. M however says that this was not at all a problem:

It was not a problem. For that we used the pit meant for garbage (*tippi*).

Selection of Method?

M decided to use condoms and did not feel like using another method:

I felt that *wanki* may be dangerous. So I thought it would be better to use Nirodh. . . . I don't want to use oral pill or *wanki*. I don't know exactly about the problems they cause. About *wanki* there are many complaints.

Some women don't get adjusted to the oral pill also. But the oral pill has fewer problems. But we want to use Nirodh.

The protection against AIDS also seems to play a role:

Recently, more information about AIDS is being given. Where was AIDS two years ago.

Telling other Women in Reproductive Ages

This respondent, unlike the other respondents, does talk with other women about spacing methods:

I tell. But these villagers are not ready for that. As I mentioned earlier they are prepared to get 3-4 children and then get operated. I told a girl here to adopt a method. But she didn't listen and also didn't try to understand.

7.4 Analysis

On the basis of these case studies, the following can be generally concluded about women who did use spacing methods:

- The women were convinced that it would be better for their health and their children's health to have some space between pregnancies;
- They thought it would be difficult to take care of more young children at a time;
- Their mother-in-law or husband was convinced it was better to space the children;
- They wanted to work and earn some money in between the births of children;
- They wanted to or were pressed to postpone their sterilization as their children were very young and they wanted to be sure that their children would survive. We call this 'new' type of 'spacing' behaviour, 'operation-postponement behaviour'.

Without the support of either the mother-in-law or the husband, it seems hardly possible for a woman to decide on her own to use spacing methods. The first case study, where C seemed to be completely in control of her pregnancies and her body, is an

exceptional case. It is remarkable that in the case studies more often mothers-in-law than husbands were informed about the use of spacing methods. Secret (not informing either the husband or the mother-in-law) use of spacing methods is definitely a possibility as the case studies indicate. A few respondents were more or less 'forced' by their mother-in-law to use spacing methods, although they were not convinced themselves. The ANM plays an important role in providing the methods. In general, personal contact with health services providers such as Anganwadi workers and ANMs seems to provide support for the use of spacing methods. The findings on the importance of contacts with health services and with socially recognized people (case study 4) give the impression that the use of spacing methods is perceived to be related to modernity.

One respondent was a 'victim' of government policy that oral pills were only provided to women with one child, and for six months only to women with two children. One other respondent had no access to the ANM as her mother-in-law did not let the ANM into her house.

Another observation is that almost none of the women in the reproductive ages advised other women in their village to use spacing methods. They felt that if their advice was followed and if something untoward happened, they would be blamed for it. It indicates that women in the reproductive ages are mainly dependent on their family-in-law, and that the peer group—in this aspect—does not play a major role. Rather, it is the family-in-law which exerts the major influence.

Quite a number of women started using spacing methods while they stayed in their mothers' place after delivery, and returned to their husband's house usually after the return of their menstruation. Most of the women used a spacing method, but did not really select a particular method.

Most women said that they did not experience major health problems as shown in Section 7.2.2. Some side-effects were mentioned, i.e. the pill causing heating, and difficulty in conceiving, but it seems that these women value the effectiveness of spacing methods, i.e. not getting pregnant, more than the possible negative side-effects. It is also remarkable that the few

women who did complain about side-effects, were also the women who used spacing methods not on their initiative but due to their mother-in-law's initiative.

7.5 Summary and Discussion

The findings in this chapter indicate that sterilization is well known, well accepted and overall practised by women in the research area. Most respondents heard about sterilization through interpersonal contacts, which—in comparison to spacing methods—is an indication of the widespread knowledge and acceptance of sterilization in the society. Sometimes, women who intend to get sterilized postpone it to the next delivery: they want to have either one (more) son or one (more) daughter or their health status is too poor to undergo an operation. Or, sometimes they want to ensure that the children will survive. In other instances, family members, husbands, mothers-in-law and mothers do not want respondents to get sterilized at that particular moment. However, in general, sterilization is accepted and is a real option for women to consider: they plan beforehand whether and when to have a sterilization, relating it to the number of children, and sons and daughters. Sterilization is thought to have some side-effects: general weakness, pain in the stomach and waist and back. However, the side-effects are not so disagreeable that women avoid sterilization. Obviously, the advantages of sterilization, i.e. to limit the children and avoid pregnancies, outweigh the disadvantages of negative health effects. One reason for the low use of spacing methods is the preference for the definitive nature of sterilization.

Regarding spacing methods, the picture is completely different. More than half of the women had heard about Copper-T and the oral pill, while less than 20 per cent had heard about condoms. The responses indicate that respondents indeed have heard about a method but it appears that they do not really *know* what the method is about, how it works, where to get it, etc. The data indicate that information on how spacing methods actually work is highly needed. Also men appear to have hardly any knowledge

about spacing methods, including condoms which they associate mainly with extramarital sex. Men contend that ANMs visit only the women and children, which leaves them out of the equation when it comes to knowledge about contraceptives.

Compared to sterilization, female respondents had heard relatively more often about spacing methods through the health services, especially the ANM. NGOs play a minor role, in general, but in particular villages the FPAI provides information and creates awareness.

The attitude towards sterilization is positive. Spacing methods on the other hand are less acceptable and the (hearsay) negative health effects play an important role. In other words, attitudes are not supportive of the use of spacing methods. Women mentioned weakness, white discharge, heating effect, as negative side-effects of the pill. Many women said that spacing methods 'do not suit their body': because they have to work hard, they cannot afford any side-effect caused by a spacing method. According to health personnel, women relate all their health problems to either sterilization or to spacing methods, although the problems may have existed earlier. The perceived health effects of spacing methods seem to be strongly related to the general health status of women in the research area (see Chapter 8 for general health status of women).

Women said that they discussed sterilization, Copper-T and oral pill predominantly with their husbands and mothers. In contrast, the mothers-in-law play a minor role in these discussions. This is interesting as the case studies indicate that the mothers-in-law influence decisions about whether or not to undergo sterilization or to use a spacing method.

Overall, the respondents were of the opinion that husbands, mothers-in-law and mothers would not agree to their using spacing methods. The normative beliefs are thus also not supportive of spacing behaviour.

Respondents, once they know the methods and where to get them, indicate that it is not difficult to go to the providers and ask for the methods. Note that all methods are provided for free by the ANM and government services. Costs of contraceptives do not seem to be a real obstacle for usage: control

beliefs are supportive of use of spacing methods.

Taking a close look at the decision processes of the few women who did use a spacing method, it seems that these women use spacing methods because they:

- were convinced that it would be better for their health and their children's health to have some time between pregnancies;
- thought it would be difficult to take care of several young children at the same time;
- had mothers-in-law/husbands who were convinced it was better to space the children;
- wanted to work and earn some money in between the birth of children;
- wanted or were 'forced' to postpone a sterilization as their children were still too young, and their survival uncertain.

Without the support of either the mother-in-law or the husband, it seems hardly possible for a woman to make her own decision to use spacing methods. More often mothers-in-law rather than husbands were informed about the use of a spacing method. The ANM plays an important role in providing the methods. The women who used a spacing method said they did not advise other women in the village to use them; they were afraid of being blamed if something went wrong. It indicates that women in the reproductive ages are mainly dependent on their family-in-law and that the peer group does not play a major role in this aspect. Chapter 9 elaborates on the status of women in different stages of the reproductive career.

Quite a number of women started using spacing methods when they stayed in their mothers' place after delivery, and before returning to their husband's house. Most of them started using these methods after the return of menstruation. Surprisingly, most women who used spacing methods said that they did not face major health problems. Some side-effects were mentioned, i.e. the pill causing heating, difficulty in conceiving again, but it seems that women who use spacing methods appreciate the effect-

iveness, i.e. not becoming pregnant, more than the possible negative side-effects.

NOTE

1. For details about health effects of tubectomy and laparoscopy, please see the interim report (Hutter et al., 2002).

8

Health Status of Women in the Reproductive Career

Chapter 7 which examined the beliefs and perceptions about spacing methods and sterilization identified attitudinal and normative beliefs as influencing spacing behaviour of women. Especially the perceived negative health effect of spacing methods was given as a reason for not using the oral pill or Copper-T. Weakness; pain in the hands, legs, back and stomach; white discharge; and heat in the body were some of the symptoms reported. Many women also said that they did not use spacing methods as they were unsuitable for them; since they have to work, they cannot afford to contend with additional health problems than those already faced. The perceived negative health effects of spacing methods thus outweigh a possible positive effect, which is to defer pregnancy. From the feedback gathered, a recurrent theme is the importance of the general health status of women.

When the women were asked in the in-depth interviews what their most important health problems were, time and again the same list of problems surfaced: *hasi may* (literally, vulnerable body), i.e. the vulnerable period after delivery, menarche and abortion. *Hasi may* after delivery and abortion have been dealt with in an earlier research (Hutter, 1994). Here, we elaborate on the event of first menstruation (Section 8.1), relating relevant health issues in *hasi may* after delivery and abortion to *hasi may* after first menstruation. In addition, we describe other aspects of the first menstruation: the existing rules about pollution and segregation (Section 8.1.1) and the concept of *arishna may* (Section 8.1.2). Section 8.2 discusses the rules about pollution and other health aspects regarding menstruation in general.

In addition, most women mentioned that they suffer from pain in their hands and legs, stomach and waist, as well as pain in their whole body. Also, white discharge (*bili muttu*) and general weakness are major problems for all women. All these symptoms seem to be interrelated (see Section 8.3).

Some older women with whom we discussed women's health problems in the villages said that nowadays cancer has become a health concern.

> It is said that cancer of *samsara* (vagina) is more common among women. Among men throat cancer is more common. Recently we have been hearing about *koosina cheela* and sometimes the cancer affects it. In that case it has to be removed.

Koosina cheela literally means 'bag of the child', namely the uterus. Section 8.4 elaborates on the knowledge of women and men about their body and the reproductive system.

The survey and in-depth interviews indicated some other related health issues. The survey data include women who had induced abortions by using so-called abortion tablets, further discussed in Section 8.5. In addition, the in-depth interviews indicated that quite a number of women have a very long first birth interval and clearly have problems conceiving again. Section 8.6 deals with the problems of conception experienced by women in the villages.

In the discussion, perceived reproductive and general health status and perceived etiology, cultural schemas (see Chapter 2) on health, illness and reproduction, which motivate reproductive health behaviour of women can be identified. In Section 8.7, we elaborate on these cultural schemas identified (in Chapters 6, 7 and 8), namely the cultural schemas of *hasi may*, purity and pollution, and heating and cooling.

8.1 Menarche

In this section, we describe health issues, customs and rules at the time of a girl's first menstruation, especially rules of segregation and pollution (Section 8.1.1) and the health concept of *hasi may* or *arishina may*. The information, gathered through in-depth interviews, refers both to the past personal experiences of women

(who are now in the reproductive ages) and to the present behaviour expected of young girls.

8.1.1 POLLUTION AND SEGREGATION

According to the women, for the first five days after the onset of the first menstruation, a girl is segregated (sitting apart) from the rest of her family. She is literally said to 'sit outside' (*horage kuditaale*). In reality it means that the girl sits in a corner of a room, or in a separate room of the house. Often a curtain is put up in order to protect her from negative influences, either from other people, the evil eye (*dristhi*) or evil spirits (*gaali*, *deva* or *butta*). A Jain respondent explained the custom:

> Usually the girl sits in the corner of a room in the house. A curtain is put up there to cover that place, to avoid evil effect on the girl caused by the arrival of different people. People come with dust on their feet and sometimes there will be the effect of *gaali*. So to avoid it, we put a curtain. People sometimes pass through the cemetery and dirty roads. Even if they wash their legs before entering the house, this much care must be taken.

Gaali literally means wind, but here it means evil spirit. The concept is explained in more detail later.

A girl who has reached menarche has to sit in the corner and should not move around in the house. She is considered to be polluting (*mailige*, *holi*) and should not touch anything or anyone and also should not be touched:

> We were not allowed either to move freely inside the house or to go outside. We had to sit in one place.

and

> We are not allowed to touch the vessels and also the broom. For five days we are not allowed to do any work.

Food is provided 'from a distance':

> Food is served to the girl from a distance. . . .

A few respondents said:

> We wash our plates and cups ourselves.

The only person who can touch the girl during the first five days

is the woman who provides her daily bath (head bath). Ideally, this person is the *sooderatte*, the girl's father's sister. In other cases, it can be another kin member. Some respondents were more particular and explained that there should be five women who are auspicious (*muttaides*) involved in providing baths during the first 5 days (see later, Chapter 9). During the first menstruation, the girl bathes in either the bathroom or a separate place outside the house. A cloth is used to cover the girl:

> Somebody holds a *saree* around the girl. A bath is given in the backyard.

Jains who have stricter rules about pollution carry out baths during these five days of pollution in the following way:

> A pit is dug outside to give the girl a bath. She is not allowed to use the common bathroom. First a pit is dug and that place is covered with cloth. Two wooden pieces cover the pit. The pit is meant to ensure that the water is absorbed by the earth. It should not flow on the roads. We have to sit on the wooden pieces and then we are given the bath, but from a distance. This arrangement is for five days.

Not only are baths given, some special body care is also provided:

> We have to apply coconut oil before a head bath. For five days *arishina* (turmeric) is also applied. Neem (*beevu*) is also applied.

Arishina is used in many other events in the reproductive career (see also Chapter 9). It is assumed to be an antiseptic. The custom of applying turmeric to the body of the girl who reaches menarche is related to the concept of *arishina may* (turmeric body) or *hasi may* (tender body).

The custom of segregation of the girl who reaches menarche is said to be practised by almost all religious and ethnic groups, including Muslims and the Gouli tribe. One Muslim respondent, however, makes a distinction between the custom of segregation (the girl sitting separately) and pollution:

> We do not follow this custom of pollution. Some people follow the custom of segregation, others don't.

Caste groups such as the Brahmins, Jains and Badigers (carpenters) are more particular about rules of purity and impurity, and also seem to be more particular about 'pouring water from a distance'. Harijan women also adhere to the prescribing

behaviour during menstruation. A Madar woman (sub-caste of the Harijans) explained:

> Up to five days we could not go to any room in the house. There is a feeling of *holi* (pollution).

People in the village observe the five-day period of pollution, as an Anganwadi worker explained, and do not visit the home of any girl who has reached menarche:

> If a girl has reached menarche they don't go to that house for five days. They visit only after five days, usually when *aarati* is done.

Aarati is the ceremony to remove the pollution after five days, and marks the end of the polluting period:

> . . . after five days *holi tagitari*.

Holi tagitari or *holi tegeyuvudu* means that the dirt has been removed. The house is cleaned, cow dung is applied to the floors, the bedding is washed, and the old bangles of the girl who experienced menarche are removed:

> On the fifth day after the bath all the bedding is washed.

The girl is given a bath. After removal of the pollution, a small ceremony, called the *sannu soobhana* (the small *soobhana*), is conducted. *Soobhanas* are songs recited during important events, especially events in the reproductive period. There are special *soobhanas* for events such as menarche, marriage, and the first pregnancy (*kubasa*) (see Chapter 9).

For some respondents, especially those from a poorer economic background, the whole ceremony is over after five days:

> We were very poor. . . . I sat apart, but only for five days. Then they sent me to the temple and finished the celebration. Nothing more was done.

For most respondents, however, a second ceremony, the *dodda soobhana* (big *soobhana*) was conducted, which is considered to be the most important ceremony (see Chapter 9).

8.1.2 *HASI MAY* OR *ARISHINA MAY*

Girls who reach menarche are considered to be in a state of *hasi may*, also known as *arishina may*, referring to the custom of

applying *arishina* on the body at the time of first menstruation. The period of *hasi may* is sometimes said to last for 16 days (so, up to the *dodda soobhana*). However, more often it lasts for one or two months. It depends, of course, on the socio-economic status of the household:

> After 1-2 months she is sent outside. For those who can afford it, the girl is kept at home for two months. But for those who cannot, the girl is sent to work immediately after menarche. People who can afford it keep the girl at home for three months. Otherwise they send the girl to work after 10-12 days. We stayed at home for one year.

During *arishina may*, a girl is supposed to be more vulnerable among others to evil spirits (*gaali*, *bhuta*, *devva*) and the evil eye (*driishti*). To protect her against these evil spirits, she is confined to the house and not allowed to go out:

> It is believed that after menarche, the girl is in *hasi may*. . . . She will be affected by the evil eye (*drishti*), as she looks more beautiful after menarche. That is an old belief.

and

> . . . The girl is in *hasi may* after menarche and so she is easily affected by *gaali*, etc. Therefore she should not go outside.

The concept of *gaali* is illustrated by a woman who recounted how she was affected by it during *hasi may* after delivery. Evil spirits are believed to be potent during special times of the day—when the sun is hot, the evening and the night. During these times they 'attack' people who are especially more vulnerable: girls who have reached menarche, women who are pregnant or have delivered.

> It is like the ghost. When we go out in the hot sun, we are affected. Moreover, people with fair or red skin soon are more easily affected. *Gaali* is around the evening or in the night or in the hot sun. If we go out at the time when it is there, its shadow falls on us.

She developed certain symptoms and went to a temple:

> I had severe fever and was admitted to the hospital. That didn't help. Then they took me to the temple of Karemma. There we came to know that it was the effect of *gaali*. . . . I had loose motion. Nothing of what I ate was stayed inside. I was affected by *gaali*.

It turned that the ghost of her father-in-law's brother was bothering her. She explained what she did to counter this ghost:

> He comes in my dream. . . . I put something under my pillow to avoid seeing him in my dream. . . . I keep a container of water and a broom or a *chappal* under the pillow before I sleep. Ghosts are scared of water, broom and *chappal.*

As mentioned before, the concept of *hasi may* applies to the period after menarche and after a delivery or abortion as well. Some women indicate that the two, *hasi may* at menarche and after delivery, are the same:

> *Hasi may* is the same in both cases. The girl or woman should not work during that period.

Another respondent confirmed that they indeed are the same but there are differences in duration:

> They are the same. After delivery it is said that the woman has *hasi may* for three months . . . (after menarche) . . . it is observed only for one month.

And another respondent stated that *hasi may* after delivery is more severe:

> During delivery women suffer a lot. So that *hasi may* is different from *hasi may* after menarche. Because during menarche, the suffering is less.

As a consequence, there are differences in the care provided:

> More care is essential after delivery than after menarche. During delivery there will be more loss of blood. If the woman gets good food she can recover soon and the child will get sufficient breast milk.

But special food is provided to the girl during *arishina may*, certainly during the first five days, but usually for a longer period:

> For the first five days we give them *kobri* (dried coconut), *uttatti* (dates), sugar, *shavige* (special sweet made of wheat), milk, *ghee* (clarified butter). . . usually these foods are given to the girl till the end of the celebration.

Other respondents talked about the provision of more sweets made out of wheat, milk and *jaggery* (cane sugar):

> *uppittu*, *shira*, *godi huggi* and *sakka aho.*

and

> They prepare *kobri*, *alavi*

These days they also prepare *bundi ladu*, rice and *kobri kara*.

Ladu is also a special sweet, specially prepared for women after delivery. It is energy-rich and made out of wheat and jaggery, nuts and raisins (see also *soobhana* in Chapter 9).

Other respondents said that fresh food should be given, i.e. freshly prepared food, not leftovers:

Everything was given fresh . . . food was fresh and hot.

Some respondents indicated:

Bisi bisi anna . . . beeku (hot, hot rice is needed).

So-called hard food is to be avoided:

They do not give us hard items like *rotti*.

The food items are exactly the same as those eaten or avoided by women after delivery. The different wheat preparations, with sugar, milk and dried fruits, are considered to be energy-rich and heating (*kaavu*) (see Hutter, 1994). After delivery, women are said to have lost a lot of blood which has to be restored by eating more *kaavu* food. After menarche, a similar reasoning seems to apply. On asking respondents why it is that especially these food items have to be given to a girl who reaches menarche, respondents said:

The girl has to become strong.

and

It is said to be nutritious.

and

May be to improve health and to help the girl to get children who will be healthy. The amount of blood in the body increases.

Besides the strengthening effect, some respondents are more specific and relate it to development of the waist and abdomen of the girl:

During menarche the girl will feel pain around her waist. So to avoid that more sweet is given to her. They also give *alavi* to her. That strengthens the waist. They give *alavi* to her after menarche as well as after delivery.

and

It is necessary for growth and development. Before menarche the waist area is not strong. They give all these things to strengthen her.

and

They give it because of *hasi may* and also because it gives strength. The abdomen is soft then. So, more sweet food is given.

But another respondent said that the custom has been followed for centuries:

Who knows the reason? It is practised by the elders.

On asking whether these foods are indeed considered to be heating the answers are not clear. A mother-in-law answered:

How can it have a heating effect? It helps the body to grow. It also tastes good. A mother knows when her daughter has reached menarche. She should grow well and she should be strong. So she gives all these things.

The girl who reaches menarche is thus provided with good food. It is not only her own family which provides food but also relatives and neighbours (who often are relatives also):

The neighbours send food, and also sweets.

Another respondent mentions the special role again for the maternal uncle, the *soodarmaava*:

In addition to this the relatives and neighbours also send food to the girl. They send *kadabu*, *karchikai*, etc. The *soodarmaava* must bring *kobri* and *uttatti*.

The special role of the maternal uncle (*soodarmaava*) is explained in more detail in Chapter 9.

8.2 Menstruation

In the local language Kannada, menstruation is indicated by the word *muttu* (menstruation) or described as *aulu horage kuditaale* (literally 'she is sitting outside'), which refers to the custom of segregation during menstruation, i.e. sitting outside, meaning: sitting apart from the family, not being allowed to enter the kitchen, to cook the food and so on. Also, the expression *neeru hanasak aagetri* is used to indicate menstruation. It means to pour

or sprinkle water, i.e. giving bath to the menstruating woman by another woman. Taking a head bath (*tale snaana*) is also associated with having monthly periods. A more recent expression is MC (menstrual cycle). A special expression, mentioned by a respondent, for the first menstruation after a postpartum period of amenorrhoea is *tottila muttu,* i.e. cradle menstruation. The different words and concepts reflect the several customs surrounding menstruation.

8.2.1 POLLUTION AND SEGREGATION

Segregation, because of pollution, is practised by respondents of different castes, usually the higher castes. In the research area, especially Jains, Brahmins, Panchal (craftsmen such as carpenters and blacksmiths) and Gouli practise the custom of segregation during menstruation. Within the Maratha caste, some respondents observe segregation, while others do not:

> If in a particular house there are *devaru* (Gods), then they follow this custom of *mailige* (pollution). Otherwise not. They can do anything and they can move anywhere in the house.

A Jain respondent said that she cannot cook for five days, every month:

> Menstruation is not a joyful occasion as it occurs at regular intervals. Even today, it is a sad thing for me. According to our custom we have to observe this practice of pollution for 4-5 days. My sister stays here only. She cooks and gives us food on those days. The men prepare tea, give us too and then they go out.

She further described the bath given during menstruation by another woman:

> Hot water is kept in the bathroom and somebody puts it in our jug and we take bath. Sometimes they give water in a bucket and we take bath ourselves. After the bath they sprinkle water on us (*neeru hanasak aagetri*). All this is preached in our Jain religion.

She compares the customs of her caste to those in the Maratha caste:

> But Maratha women don't practice such a thing. They take head-baths

immediately after getting their periods and then move freely in the house. What I tell you is exactly what I practise regularly, i.e. according to Jain *dharma*.

She reflects:

According to me it is not correct, what Maratha people do. To move freely around the house while having periods is not correct according to me. I have a feeling of pollution.

The custom of segregation implies that everyone in the house knows about a woman's periods. Menstruation then is not a private affair but common knowledge to the whole family. This is considered to be quite normal:

Menstruation is common for all. If we observe it within our family, what harm is there? According to our *dharma* we have to follow it. Moreover menstruation is common for all women. Only family members get to know about it . . . is a fact and nobody can control it.

Respondents talked about the advantages of segregation, i.e. they get rest for some days:

We get rest. We don't have to carry out work like cooking, etc.

Not all respondents of the higher castes are able to comply with the custom of segregation or to follow all prescriptions. Sometimes only some of the customs are followed. A common practice is to refrain from *puja* and not to take a head bath during menstruation:

In our house we don't follow it. We don't touch the god. We take a head bath immediately after we get menstruation, whether it is in the morning or in the evening. Somebody in the family gives the bath. I request my co-sister. We take head bath on all the five days to become clean or pure (*shuddha*).

Whether a respondent observes the custom of segregation often depends on her economic and social circumstances, especially on the composition of the household. One respondent from the Panchal (craftsmen) group described the following:

In our community of carpenters, during menstruation we stay segregated for four days. We don't enter the *puja* room. We don't touch anything, not even touch the water that is inside the kitchen. On the fourth day we take a

> head bath, wash our clothes, etc., and only then we enter into the kitchen and *puja* room.

Another Panchal respondent said:

> Here we do all the work. But in my *tavaru mane* we don't do any work for five days. During that period we have to sit apart. But here we are given a head bath immediately after we get menstruation.

And a woman living in a nuclear family said that she could follow the custom only when she and her husband stayed with her in-laws:

> Now I carry out all the household work. When we stayed together with the in-laws, for five days I used to be segregated. That is, I used to work outside, like washing the clothes, cleaning the vessels, bringing water in the morning and then cooking. For five days I keep my bedding separately.

Generally, the period of pollution lasts for five days. The pollution is removed by cleaning the house, washing the clothes:

> We clean the whole house with cow dung, wash the clothes and then enter the house.

Most respondents, however, keep it simple during menstruation: they do not take a head bath everyday, and bathe on their own:

> Now I take a bath first and then go inside and do every thing. We heat water and then take a bath ourselves. Sometimes they pour water on us.

and

> I apply some oil and take a head bath immediately after I get my periods. Then I go inside. Only on the first and last days we take a head-bath. On the remaining days we just bathe.

A Muslim respondent said that in her community women do not follow the rule of segregation during menstruation. They only follow it during the first menstruation.

8.2.2 BEHAVIOUR DURING MENSTRUATION

As mentioned before, women who practise segregation are not allowed to do household work and are only allowed to enter the kitchen after five days. Cooking is done by other family members.

Most women, however, do cook during these days. But none of them conducts *puja* and prepares food 'for the Gods':

> We don't even touch the food prepared to offer to the God and we don't do *puja*. But we do the cleaning of the house and also washing.

Another respondent said:

> . . . *Puja?* Impossible. Up to seven days we don't go to *puja* room and do the *puja*. On the fifth day we wash our hair and on the sixth day and seventh days we apply oil to our head and do the *puja*.

In Chapter 6, we discussed the custom of sexual abstinence during religious festivals and *puja*, as sexual relations—like menstruation and also childbirth—are considered to be polluting. Respondents mentioned they could conduct *puja* again from the fifth, sixth or seventh day after menstruation. The rule of not doing *puja* is quite clear and is also strictly followed by women.

Muslim respondents too observe some rules during menstruation:

> For five days we shouldn't touch the incense sticks. . . . We do the cooking, but we should not offer the food prepared by us during those days to God. We can do that after taking head bath.

Another Muslim respondent said that menstruating women are not allowed to light the lamp, and how this custom made her mother-in-law, who diligently noted her monthly periods, aware of her pregnancy:

> Usually elderly women observe the menstruation of other women in the house. My mother-in-law also observed my periods. When I didn't get my periods for two months she asked me. . . . On every Thursday we light the lamp for god. If I am menstruating and she asks me to light the lamp, I tell her that I can't do it. But for two months she observed that I was lighting the lamp without any interruption. So she came to know about it and asked me.

Menstruating women are also not supposed to attend special ceremonies:

> If there is a special occasion, then we tell that we have got periods. We don't do any thing until the menstruation is over. We take the menstrual dates into account before fixing the date of marriage.

All these customs make clear that menstruation is quite a public

affair, overtly indicated and observed by family and community members.

Menstruating women should not touch children as it causes children to be sick, so-called *muttu dosha*:

> If a menstruating woman touches a child that child becomes thin. Then it is believed that the child is suffering from *muttu dosha*.

and

> The children dry up (*wana*). They become very thin. Then we come to know that the child is suffering from *muttu dosha*.

Muttu dosha can affect a child up to the age of 12 years, but the effect is strongest during the first five years:

> If they are below 12 years it is not that serious a problem. But children who are below five years or infants should not be touched by a menstruating woman.

However, as one of our respondents explained: when a woman is sterilized she can touch children during menstruation, i.e. it will not lead to *muttu dosha*:

> Yes, we can touch them. We can even touch other children. Because I got operated and I can't have any more children. So, people also give their children if necessary . . . it is accepted. . . . The conception is stopped. So, it is believed that there will be no problem for children. Otherwise they can become thin.

This seems to indicate that menstruation as such is not considered to have an adverse effect on children, menstruation in a fertile woman (i.e. when she is able to conceive) is regarded as harmful.

8.2.3 HEALTH ASPECTS

In general, respondents said that they experience some general pain at the time of menstruation: a piercing sensation in the stomach, around the waist. Others talked about the feeling of heaviness in the body:

> I don't have stomach pain and all that. Only on the first day I feel pain in the waist portion (*nada novu*) and heaviness of the body (*mai vajje*), that is all.

None of the respondents described problems which could be

classified as pre-menstrual syndrome (PMS). When PMS was explained to women, none of them even recognized it. Only one respondent said:

> When the dates are nearing, then I experience problems *nada novu* (waist pain), pain in the stomach and legs. During the rest of the days, I don't have any problems. When I get these aches then I come to know and after two to three days time I get my periods. I also feel like sleeping.

It is considered good to have a regular menstruation. If it is irregular, it is believed that impure blood remains in the body, the body becomes heavy and the woman might develop an illness:

> If I get menstruation every month regularly, I feel good. Otherwise it leads to problems. I feel heaviness in the body. If it is regular it is good. If I get it regularly, the problem will be for just two days. If it is late there will be more problems.

> If it doesn't come out once a month, women will have some disease, i.e. *roga* (disease). Then blood remains in the body itself. That should not happen it must come out. If menstruation doesn't start for one or two months, then we must go to the doctor. Sometimes for the women in the villages the menstruation may stop for one year and there may not be any problem. But after that period menstruation must start at a regular interval of 20 days or one month.

One woman indicated that if her menstruation is not regular, she feels heavy and is not being able to eat:

> If I menstruate regularly every month, I feel good. The body will not be heavy. Otherwise if I don't get menstruation for 2-3 months, my body will become heavy. I experience problems similar to those in early pregnancy. I feel heavy even after eating very little and I do not feel like doing any work for one hour after meals. I feel better if I don't take food.

Related to regularity, most respondents consider heavy bleeding to be good. According to them it makes the body light:

> Heavy flow is good. The body will be light.

If the bleeding is light it is believed to lead to some illness, i.e. pain in legs and hands and body:

> It is good if there is heavy bleeding . . . it is believed like that. It is said that less bleeding leads to ill health. . . . There will be severe pain in the legs and hands and the body will ache.

and

> If there is less bleeding it leads to problems in the stomach—pain in the stomach and waist portion. There will be problems inside the stomach too.

Yet another respondent said that when the bleeding is light and blood remains in the body, a blood clot forms inside:

> It is good to have heavy bleeding. Otherwise some problems develop inside. It is said that a mass will form.

Some respondents think that women who have light bleeding during the monthly periods are anaemic:

> In a way less bleeding is good. But for good health, heavy bleeding is good, which depends upon the quantity of blood in the body. If we have less blood in our body and we are dried up (*wana*), then we have less bleeding.

and

> I am not healthy. That much blood also is not there in the body, so bleeding is less.

Also in Chapter 6, women mentioned that their period of post-partum amenorrhoea was longer because they had not enough blood in their body as a result of blood loss during delivery. Similarly, a respondent who underwent sterilization and then experienced less bleeding during menstruation explained:

> Before my operation there was more bleeding. Now it is less. . . . I feel that it is less due to less blood in the body.

Thus, the respondents think that light bleeding during menstruation is related to

- having less blood in the body;
- literally, being dried up (*wana*), i.e. having less strength and being more weak.

We return to this relationship in Section 8.7.

Heavy bleeding is considered to be good as it removes all the dirt inside the body:

> I have heavy bleeding since the beginning. Some women say that heavy bleeding is good. All the dirt should go out of the body.

A herbal medicine (*gavati*) can be taken to induce heavier bleeding:

During menstruation when bleeding was less regular, I took a *gavati* medicine. It was some green juice. We had to go there on first day of menstruation itself, on empty stomach. Early in the morning we have to go there and drink that juice. . . . Since I took that medicine the bleeding is in correct quantity.

So, light bleeding is not considered to be good, and heavy bleeding is considered to cleanse the body. However, too heavy a bleeding is also not considered to be good. A mother-in-law said:

One should not have heavy bleeding. It reduces body strength. We have to work hard. Heavy bleeding leads to weakness. If it is medium that is good. . . . If blood is lost in greater quantity, then waist pain starts. There will be pain in the hands and legs. The body will have strength only if it has the required quantity of blood. If there is energy in the body, a person can work hard and for a longer time. It depends upon one's body constitution . . . there may be heavy bleeding or light.

and

Heavy bleeding also leads to problems. If there is heavy bleeding there will be pain in the hands and legs and one cannot walk.

In conclusion, as a respondent expressed:

Moderate bleeding is good for health. If bleeding is heavy, we don't feel comfortable (*bejaru*). Our body will ache due to heavy bleeding. If the bleeding is too light, then it is said that some tumours will form in the stomach. That is also not good. So it is good to have moderate bleeding.

Another respondent related heavy bleeding to the extra care to be taken:

We go out for work and if there is heavy bleeding we can't change the cloth. We go out in the morning, we come back home in the evening. We can't change the cloth in between. Therefore I feel that less bleeding is good.

Women use cloth during menstruation and wash it either in the tank near the village, or at home:

We use cloth. We wash it, dry it and use it again. We go to the tanks or lakes to bathe. There we wash and dry the cloth. We have to do our work ourselves, but we have to do it secretly. How to show it to others? As far as possible we try to do it secretly.

On asking the respondents what women can do if their menstruation is late, some respondents are very clear and direct and

mention that they can have abortion tablets or injections (see Section 8.5):

> They take tablets or injections from the ANM to start menstruation.

In earlier times, women used home remedies in order to bring on their menstruation when it was delayed. A common method was eating food which was heating (*ushna* or *kaavu*):

> Earlier it is said that women used to eat papaya and *alavi*. . . . Yes (it has a heating effect). But nowadays women go directly to the doctor. They don't use such things anymore.

The interpreter said that it is commonly known that eating *yellu* (sesame) and *kachu* (used in *pan*), or hard physical work will lead to an early menstruation. These are considered to have heating qualities.

In order to get a clear picture, we inquired further about whether there is a relationship between menstruation and items which cause heating. Many respondents said there is no link between the two. One respondent explained, however:

> No. It is not heating in a regular course. But whenever menstruation comes early or late, then only people say that it is due to heating.

This means that if there is excess heat in the body, menstruation will start earlier. And if menstruation is late, heating items can be taken to induce menstruation. The finding in Chapter 6, that the heating qualities of the oral pill causes more bleeding is explicable in this context.

Some respondents indicated that they sometimes deliberately postponed their menstruation—to be able to attend a function—by taking tablets:

> I took tablets. During the festival of Mahanavami, there is *puja* in our house. So at that time I took those tablets. For other festivals I don't take.

and

> Generally women take tablets to postpone the menstruation.

Do respondents have any idea how menstruation comes about? Most of them do not have any idea (see also Section 8.4). One respondent explained:

A girl reaches menarche around the age of 14; 16 years is the upper limit. The girl is said to be at the proper age. When the uterus starts growing, menstruation starts. As a rule it starts. . . . After reaching the age of menarche blood will flow from the uterus. It collects there and comes out.

8.3 Common Health Problems of Women: Weakness Syndrome

As indicated in the Introduction, following *hasi may* women in the villages identified the following other common health problems: pain in the hands and legs, stomach and waist, weakness and white discharge. The symptoms are very much related to each other. The root lies in women's general weakness.

8.3.1 Pains, White Discharge and General Weakness

A very common complaint of the women in the villages is the pain felt in the hands and legs, and in the stomach or waist: 'pain in the waist portion, pain in the legs'; 'stomach ache, waist pain, pain in the legs and hands'; 'pain in the legs, backache, headache'.

The last respondent related the problems to the heavy workload for women in the village:

Women in the villages have to take care of children, finish the housework and go out for work, travel, etc. This leads to such problems.

A Gouli respondent added:

There will be four to five children at home. She must cook for them and she has to fetch water. Bringing water, wood, grass for cattle . . . go to the forest, work hard, collect seeds from forest.

An Ayurvedic physician in one of the villages, relates the common problems of pain in the hands and legs to the concept of heating (*kaavu*, *ushna*), and recommends that women eat cooling (*tampu)* food such as *halu* (milk), *majjige* (buttermilk) and *mosaru* (curds). This is not only because these food items have cooling qualities and compensate the heating, but also because they are nutritious.

What do women do to relieve the pain in their hands and legs? In general, respondents believe strongly in tablets and injections. However, they can hardly afford them, as the costs are too high:

If we go out in the rain we suffer from cold or fever; we take rest for two days. We can't afford the injections due to lack of money and lack of time. We buy Novalgin tablets from the shop. . . . A doctor comes here. Sometimes we go to city D, and sometimes we go to city A. If the problem is severe we go there. Just for headache, etc., we don't go to the doctor. We can't afford that expenditure, going by bus and the charge of the medicine. We get the tablets in the shops for 50 paise or Re. 1. We take one or two tablets and feel better.

Pains in the hands, legs, stomach, waist, and back might be a sign of general weakness and deficiencies in nutrition.

In addition, white discharge (*bili muttu*, literally white menstruation) is a very commonly experienced health problem for women in the villages:

It is common. Almost 90 per cent of women have such a problem or a variation in menstrual dates and white discharge.

and

It is found in many women. If the problem is severe, it is said that the strength will go to waste.

and

It is said that all women have that problem.

An ANM describes different types of *bili muttu*:

There are different colours: red, brown, light pink, black, etc. If they complain about such things, then we tell them to consult the doctor. . . . Reasons may be different. It may be a sign of cancer too. Sometimes there will be itching and burning sensation. . . .

Respondents, only made a distinction is between *kempu muttu* (red menstruation) which we first interpreted as common menstruation, and *bili muttu*, or white discharge. However, one respondent specified:

Sometimes the discharge will be white and sometimes red. There will also be pain in the waist portion, legs and hands.

Other specifications from respondents were:

Before I conceived, I had such a problem . . . the flow was like curd. It had that consistency.

and

(White discharge . . .) seems like my bones are coming out of my body.

Remarkably, many women relate white discharge to other reproductive events and indicated that they started to have problems of *bili muttu* after either a delivery or sterilization:

My problem started only after the operation. Many people say like that it is related to the operation.

and

Now I have problems like white discharge, after the delivery of this girl. Earlier I didn't have any problem. . . . I don't know what is the reason. Almost every day I have white discharge.

Also the use of Copper-T, as indicated in Chapter 6, is related to white discharge:

I have heard that by using Copper-T *bili muttu* will start.

Another woman relates white discharge to her menstruation:

After menstruation, when bleeding becomes less, then discharge starts.

And very commonly, it is linked to sexual contacts:

When we have sex, I get that problem for two days.

A very clear relationship is made between white discharge and weakness. The two respondents who related the discharge to delivery and sterilization later stated that it was actually caused by weakness:

Many people say that it starts due to weakness. Nobody tells anything other than this.

The respondents thus make a link between weakness—either due to operation or delivery—and white discharge. Another woman mentioned:

Another point is that it starts due to heavy work.

Thus, *bili muttu* and the other common health problems among women in the village, i.e. pain in hands and legs, stomach and waist, and weakness are all related. The causal link is not always clear:

The other problems related to *bili muttu* . . . women say that *nada novu* (waist pain), *kai-kalu novu* (pain in hand and legs) are common.

and

I have waist pain and white discharge. The problem is very severe. When I have that problem I experience severe pain in the legs, hands and waist.

Others attributed health problems to be the cause of white discharge:

If the woman has some disease in the body she will have problems like headache. Sometimes after sexual intercourse there is white discharge. Health problems like waist pain are due more to *bili muttu*. People will be talking about it: after having sex women may experience *bili muttu*. It is a belief. Some women say that the pain in legs, waist portion, weakness and lack of blood lead to *bili muttu*.

And again others stated that the health problems are the consequences of *bili muttu*:

Weakness and waist pain. We feel as if the legs have lost this strength. I can't lift heavy items. I can't walk a long distance.

Another common perception is that white discharge is caused by heat (*kaavu*):

It is caused by heat also.

and

When I consulted the doctor, I was told that it was caused due to heat.

The Ayurvedic physician indeed also related the white discharge to heat and weakness (*ashekti*, *wana*). In addition, he also thought that the problem of general weakness meant that there was less blood in the body. This is a common idea because the women also indicated that they had less blood in their body when they were weak. The Ayurvedic physician related having less blood to less heat (*kaavu*) in the body.

An earlier case study reported white discharge to be related to sexual relationships. Sexual intercourse is often classified as heating. According to an ANM, smoking and alcohol are also considered to be extremely heating. So, if sexual intercourse takes place while alcohol and cigarettes are taken, even more heat is created and this heat is passed on to women, leading to white discharge. The ANM added the lack of hygiene as a reason for the common problem of *bili muttu:*

We don't find cleanliness among them. They don't even bathe daily.

On asking respondents what they do when they had white discharge, one of them said that she did not do anything:

I am shy to go to the doctor. Any way we have to die one day. So I haven't cared for it.

Some herbal medicines (*gavati*) can be taken:

They eat white hibiscus . . . they fry it in *ghee* and then eat it . . . the problem of white discharge becomes less. The quantity is reduced. It is taken as medicine because it reduces the white discharge.

As white discharge is considered to be due to heat, we asked whether there is a belief that the discharge occurs due to heat and this white hibiscus has cooling effect. While a respondent disagreed, an older respondent confirmed the cooling effect of the herbs.

8.4 Knowledge and Perceptions about the Reproductive System

We asked our respondents whether they have any idea about their reproductive organs, what they look like, how they function and so on. It was quite a difficult question. In general, we related it to the questions on menstruation, *bili muttu* and childbirth, and asked whether women knew where menstruation comes from, where the child grows (*koosina cheela* = literally bag for the child; the uterus).

It was clear that most respondents do not have any knowledge. The typical answers were:

No. I don't know anything.

or

God knows about it. He has created it and he knows about it.

and

I don't understand and I also don't think that much. I don't know much.

and

No, I haven't heard. We don't even go outside. We don't go anywhere. We also haven't heard anything about such things.

Some respondents know a bit more:

> I don't know why it (menstruation) happens: It will be there till the women grow older, say the villagers. Only during pregnancy, women don't get menstruation.

and

> It (menstruation) starts every month. It is natural. . . . It goes on for almost half of our life span. Now my mother-in-law doesn't menstruate.

Another respondent said that menstruation comes from the stomach (*hotte*):

> It is from the stomach (*hotte*) only. . . . I have heard (about *kusina cheela*). But I don't know anything aboutit.

The word stomach (*hotte*) is generally used for the whole lower part of the trunk. In an earlier research (Hutter, 1994), we found that pregnancy is indicated as women 'being with a stomach'. A tubectomy is mentioned as 'the stomach has been cut', an inducted abortion as 'the stomach has been washed', a spontaneous abortion as 'the stomach has stopped'.

The answers given indicate that women hardly have any knowledge about their body and about their reproductive organs. However, some women do have knowledge but express it in their own words and ways. A respondent, in answering the question where menstruation comes from, said:

> It comes from the place where the child comes out.

Another word used for vagina is *udibayi*. The *udi*, as described in more detail in Chapter 9, is the front part of the *saree* which, in many ceremonies such as menarche, marriage, pregnancy and naming ceremony, is filled with grains and fruits. It also refers to the lap: The word *bayi* means mouth. We interpret the word *udibayi* thus to mean the mouth of the *udi*. On asking one of the respondents about this interpretation, however, she explained:

> They say that the *koosina cheela* has not come to the *udibayi* . . . it is just called that way.

On asking whether there is a link with the *udi*, she says:

> No. That is different. We say the child's head does not come to the *udibayi*. That *udi* is different from this *udi* or *samsara*.

Samsara is another word used by women for vagina. Literally, it means the whole world.

(The place, from where the child comes out . . .) . . . is called *samsara*.

On asking whether the word *yoni* is also used, she explains:

Usually the word *samsara* is used. Some may call it as the place from where urine comes (*kalmadi jjaga*). But the most used word is *samsara*.

Kalmadi jjaga is the urinary tract, and is here confused with the vagina. In the interviews among men *samsara* is also used to indicate the penis.

Another respondent clearly pointed out that menstruation comes from the *samsara* and that children grow in the *koosina cheela*:

(menstruation comes) from *samsara*. Menstruation does not come from *koosina cheela*. The babies grow there. When the *koosina cheela* is operated on the bleeding becomes less.

Earlier we translated *koosina cheela* as uterus. However, it does not seem to be only the uterus itself, but literally 'the bag that holds the foetus'. On answering a question what people say if there are some problems during delivery, and the labour pains have stopped, a respondent says:

They say that the *koosina cheela* has not come to the *udibayi*.

One mother-in-law who only recently became a birth attendant and had a training in a hospital in Dharwad explained further:

If the child doesn't come out soon, it is said that the *koosina cheela* has not come out. Sometimes it is said that delivery was conducted by tearing it. If the *koosina cheela* is stiff, the child cannot move its hands and legs at all. It is not a common thing, it happens only when our time is not good. It is said that the delivery was conducted by tearing the *koosina cheela*. . . . It is known after the child comes out. How can it be known when it is inside? The child sits inside the *koosina cheela* like a ball. When it comes along with the cover, the *soolagitti* has to tear it and then the child comes out and cries. *Koosina cheela* has a cover. We tear that cover.

Later on in the interview, referring to delivery, she said:

We say the pains have stopped or the child is not in the *marga*.

Marga literally means tract.

Some respondents have knowledge, which is more related to the biomedical model:

A girl reaches menarche around the age of 14; 16 years is the limit. The girl is said to be at the proper age. When the uterus starts growing, menstruation starts. As a rule it starts. After reaching the age of menarche blood will flow from the uterus. It collects there and comes out. If menstruation doesn't come once a month, women will have some disease, i.e. *roga* (a disease). Then the blood remains in the body. But that should not happen. It must come out. If there is no menstruation for one or two months, then we must go to the doctor. Sometimes for the women in the villages the menstruation may stop for one year. There may not be any problem. But even after that period menstruation must start at the regular interval of 20 days or one month.

Another woman, educated, stated even more precisely:

In the family planning office they had given the information. Women in the villages usually don't know anything about it. But those who get some information from the doctor, etc., know about it. . . . I don't remember. It was said that there are egg-like things in the stomach. They come to the *koosina cheela* and then the menstruation starts.

An ANM tells how she educates women about their body:

We show them diagrams. We show them a picture of the uterus. Then we show them the route a child takes during delivery. Then we talk about ovaries.

She often relates it to the agricultural cycle:

If we tell them in a way they know they can understand it easily. We compare it to the sowing in the fields. The ovaries release an egg every month. We explain it to them in terms of sowing in the field. The semen from the male enters the uterus from another side. When it unites with the egg released by the ovaries, conception takes place. . . . They laugh when we show them the pictures. They also laugh when they see the illustration of a vasectomy operation. Only some women understand what we say. Those who are educated like us keep quiet. Others keep on laughing.

After asking respondents whether they knew about periodic abstinence (see also Chapter 6), we subsequently asked them when conception takes place. Almost all respondents had no idea, but were eager to know more about it. One respondent expressed some ideas about when conception takes place, but confused the infertile and fertile days. Some knowledge about fecundity is

present in the *Panchanga*, the astrological book consulted by villagers (see also Chapter 9). It states that the most fecund period is between 5 and 16 days after menstruation. If the counting starts from the last day of menstruation, and assuming that menstruation lasts for five days, it is actually almost similar to the biomedical model. The astrologer whom we interviewed said that the *Panchanga* includes several ideas about periodic abstinence, or when it is best to have sexual relations in order to conceive. He read the *Panchanga* to us, indicating that couples could even determine the sex of their child:

> If they have sex on sixth day after menstruation it is said that the conception is definite. Till 4th-5th day it is not advised. Conception is said to be definite on 8th, 10th, 12th, 14th and 16th days. . . . Here it is also said that except for some bad days and *nakshatras*, if the husband and wife have sex on even days till the 16th day after menstruation, they will get a male child. If they have sex on odd days, they will have a female child. A woman can conceive between 5th and 16th days after menstruation.

The interviews among men revealed that they have varied perceptions and knowledge about the relationship between sex and pregnancy and how life is formed in the woman's womb. They also differ in terms of their understanding of the fertile period during the woman's menstrual cycle. Almost all men said that pregnancy is related to sexual intercourse, but how exactly conception takes place is not known to any. Their understanding of the human reproductive system and reproduction is very different from the biomedical model. Some feel that the women too have something similar to the *indriya* (semen) that the men have, and the joining of the two leads to pregnancy. Some think that the woman has a flower-like organ inside the vagina that opens up during menstruation, and if the man's semen falls on it, it automatically closes and forms a bag in which a child grows. The idea about the fertile period in a woman's menstrual cycle is completely opposite to what the biomedical model suggests. For instance, some men reported that if one wants a child, he should have sex during menstruation when the vagina has opened up. Most men felt that 5-8 days after the first day of menstruation is the most fertile period to have children. Many reported the fifth day as the most ideal.

8.5 Induced Abortions

The survey indicates that of all pregnancy outcomes, 0.6 per cent are induced abortions (see Chapter 5). An ANM confirmed that the number of induced abortions is indeed low in the villages:

> Such cases are not common in villages. They decide to get that child delivered and after that to get operated. Some think why should we get it removed when there is pregnancy and some think of getting it removed.

Another respondent:

> They prefer to deliver that child and then think of a permanent method to stop it. The idea of removing it is very rare in villages. They think it is dangerous and so get operated soon.

An ANM tells:

> There are very few cases. In the past, such cases used to be more.

But if induced abortions are conducted, women will surely not openly talk about it. One respondent who told us that she had an induced abortion, had it carried out without her husband's and mother-in-law's knowledge. On asking what women can do if they have an unwanted pregnancy, they said that they could use the so-called abortion tablets:

> In that situation some women may take tablets to get it out. . . .

In the next section, we discuss these so-called abortion tablets, while Section 8.5.2 deals with other methods thought to induce abortions.

8.5.1 Abortion Tablets

On pursuing further about the so-called abortion tablets, e.g. where they can be bought, how they work, a respondent explained:

> They can go to the hospital and take tablets to get it removed. Otherwise they continue the pregnancy. Along with the tablets, an injection is also given. And pregnancy will not continue. We get the tablets in Haliyal. . . . Daily two tablets for a period of seven days. . . . First they give two injections and then they give tablets. . . . The foetus comes out in seven days. . . . It has a lot of side-effects. The body dries up (*wana*). Immediately after seven days the foetus drops out.

Initially, we thought that these abortion tablets are abortion pills. However, that seemed too expensive for the villages, as a general practitioner in Dharwad indicated. An ANM explained later that these tablets are actually not really abortion tablets, but tablets that are used as a kind of pregnancy test:

Earlier some tablets were given for testing. But later that company closed down. But to my knowledge no such tablets are used nowadays. Once when we had asked the doctor about it, he said that nothing happens when the tablets are given. The only means for an abortion is D&C (Dilatation and Curettage) or MTP (Medical Termination of Pregnancy). Some women say that the abortion took place due to such and such tablets. But officially such a tablet is not available.

Another ANM explained that these tablets are EP-Forte tablets:

Actually it is for pregnancy testing. Its name is EP-Forte. It doesn't suit some women and when they take it menstruation starts. . . . It is used to test whether a woman is pregnant or not. But they think that the pills are meant for abortion. . . . They wait for eight days after the tablet is given. If menstruation starts within eight days, it means that there is no pregnancy. Otherwise it means that there is pregnancy.

She added:

We are not allowed to give those tablets. They have to go to a doctor. They take it because they know that it does not suit everyone. So if they want an abortion, they like to take them. . . . They go to a doctor and get the prescription sometimes. . . . The problem arises when they are unmarried.

8.5.2 OTHER ABORTION METHODS: HEATING ITEMS

Besides the so-called abortion tablets, there are other methods to induce an abortion. A respondent said that Anacin tablets (against headache) can be used to induce an abortion:

Usually women take the tablets, especially the Anacin tablet.

In general, allopathic medicines are classified as heating (*kaavu*) and if used during pregnancy they might induce a (spontaneous) abortion. A respondent explained this heating effect:

I was one and half months pregnant and I didn't know about it yet. I had severe headache and I took an Anacin tablet. After four to five days, it got aborted. Once again I had taken it. Then also the result was the same. Since

then my periods have became irregular. I took it only for headache. I did not know that I was pregnant.

Another respondent mentioned heating foods used earlier to induce an abortion: papaya and *alavi*:

In the past, it is said that women were using them. . . . They used to eat papaya and *alavi*. . . . Yes (*alavi* has a heating effect). Now such things don't have any effect . . . nowadays women go directly to the doctor. They don't use such things anymore.

Heating items thus do not only trigger menstruation (see above), but also induce abortion. Earlier research found that heating items were also used to hasten labour for a fast delivery. A mother-in-law mentioned that in earlier times indeed herbal methods were used to induce an abortion. Actually, she took the herbal medicine (*gavati*) herself:

There was *gavati* medicine for that. I felt I had enough children and took *gavati* medicine. I wanted to get rid of that child. . . . Maybe in the fourth or fifth month (I took the medicine). But it didn't have any effect upon me. I haven't told about it to anybody here. Only now I am telling it. An old man gave me that medicine. It was green. I took it, but it didn't work.

The medicine did not work for her, she believes, as the *gavati* medicine works only in instances of illegal pregnancies:

He told me it was so because mine was not an illegal pregnancy. That person told me that if it were an illegal pregnancy, the child would have died. These days young people do 'love' each other. They are not married and they do it secretly. If it were so, it would have died. But mine is a sacred relationship of husband and wife. That is why the child remained in the stomach, even after taking the medicine.

Induced abortion thus seems to be mainly associated with pre-marital pregnancies.

8.6 Problems in Conception

In the in-depth interviews, several respondents indicated that their first child was born late because they had difficulties in conceiving. Also in Chapter 7, several respondents expressed the fear that after the use of the oral pill they might not be able to conceive again. In this section, a few case studies are presented

about respondents who, at the time of the interview, had not been able to conceive after having given birth to one or more children. The focus is especially on perceptions of these women and the reactions in their immediate social environment. In addition, we present some case studies of women who got children in spite of having problems conceiving. Remedies against infertility are discussed as well.

One of the respondents, who was not able to conceive for more than five years after having given birth to two daughters, said that people said that she had become a stone (*kallu*), i.e. not able to conceive:

> She . . . became *kallu*.

Her family wanted her to have one more child, a son:

> They want a boy. Now I have two daughters. After marriage they will go to their husband's houses. Who will be there to look after us in old age? They argue like this. But I haven't yet conceived. Everybody wants me to have one more child. So I have to wait. If I conceive let it be a boy or a girl, that doesn't make any difference. After that I will think of operation. I consulted some ANM and doctors. They also told me not get operated yet because I have only two daughters and no son. If I get a son, then I can get operated.

However, in her opinion, it does not really matter:

> These two daughters are enough for me. I don't have any longing for a son. Actually I don't want to have either a son or a daughter. It is better if I remain like this.

Another (a Muslim) respondent whose first son was born three years after marriage and who has not been able to conceive for the past 10 years, explained that she and her family do not consider it to be a problem. She referred several times to God and fate:

> The elders in the house said that if I had one more child, girl or boy, the first son would have company. . . . What is there to feel? We have to accept if God gives. Otherwise I don't expect anything. I accept one more child if God gives. If we have luck, we will get one more child. Otherwise people will say that she has only one son.

Her husband had the same opinion:

> He . . . also says not to take pills or anything like that. If the conception

takes place it is good. If there is no conception that is also fine. If a second child is written in our fate, we will get it.

She felt, however, that it would be good for her son to enjoy the company of a sister or brother:

It is good if the first child has company. When we see sometimes other people quarrelling, I feel that it is better to have two. But it is God who gives.

When we asked about the reactions of other people in the village, she said:

They may be teasing behind my back, but not in front of me.

On asking whether she was doing anything special in order to conceive:

Nobody told me anything. Anyway it is late. God may give or may not. It is all written in our fate. Some people get a child every year, even if they don't want one. What can we do? Nothing of that sort was told.

Also, women who—in their opinion—had their first pregnancy late considered conception to be beyond control:

the God should give.

and

I feel that let it happen any time, if it is written in our fate.

and

People who have children in their fate get children, otherwise nothing can help them.

Unlike the respondents just described, others tried remedies to solve the problems of conceiving. The different possibilities available indicate the overall importance of women having children. Praying is one of the possibilities to solve infertility or subfecundity, as a (Muslim) respondent, indicated:

Only thing is we had prayed to God. I prayed to him to give me a child. My father-in-law also went to pray to God. . . .

A Maratha respondent delivered her first child after nine years of her marriage, only after she made offerings to a Muslim God:

During the ninth year I got my first child. They gave *udi* (part of worship,

see Chapter 9) to the Muslim God *Alladevaru.* Within one year after the *udi*, I got my first child. . . . Within a year after that I got another child. One of my co-sisters had tried and she had got a child. So we went thereafter that.

Similarly, a respondent who complained that no conception took place until three years after her marriage said that prayers help. Interestingly enough, like the case study just described, the prayers were addressed to a Muslim Goddess:

Near my *tavaru mane* there is a Muslim goddess, Bea Phatima. I was advised to give her *udi* after menstruation. I gave her *udi* on fifth or sixth day after menstruation. That same month I conceived. By the time of the fair I was three months pregnant. The *udi* which we keep there will be as fresh as it was on the day when we brought it there, if everything goes well.

After the birth of her child, she thanked the Goddess and the temple for the blessing. Her parents presented a fluorescent tube to the temple:

I also fulfilled what I wanted to give to the temple. I wanted to give a fluorescent tube and I gave it to them . . . my parents gave that. The practice is that only the *tavaru mane* (mothers' place) people should give it. . . . Within three years of giving the first *udi* I was pregnant and I had got two children in total. The effect of that *udi* can be seen within three years. . . .

If a conception does not take place within three years, there are other things that still can be done. According to the respondent:

If within three years no change takes place, then they think of getting a special thread around the hand. If a woman does not have children in her life at all, then nothing can help her, neither the *udi* nor the thread. If she does not get children after trying both, then they have to give up hope. . . . It is a red thread, with special power. The priest there ties it . . . (Gods are) . . . one is Bea Phatima, and another I don't remember the name. They are husband and wife.

The Gouli respondents said that couples who are unable to conceive go to a special temple in Pandharpur:

They had been to Pandharpur and got one son after nine daughters.

In addition, in the Gouli hamlet, three stones, brought from the forest area where the Gouli originally lived, can be worshipped by people who cannot have children:

If those who don't have children ask for those God stones, and worship them they will definitely get children.

In addition, there is a custom that women have to visit a special tree and do a *puja*:

Usually by going around the *patri* tree five times every day, they will get children. They go to the tree on particular days. They take *akki kalu* (rice and grain) and incense sticks and go rounds around the tree five times. Then they leave the *akki kalu* there and light the incense sticks. They do *namaskara* to the tree. On the last day they are told to offer coconut and banana to that tree. Then they come back home and give them to other children.

As discussed in Chapter 9, *akki kalu*, i.e. rice and grains, is used in several ceremonies during wedding ceremonies and can be interpreted as a symbol of fertility.

Social pressure to conceive after marriage is definitely present. On asking a respondent what her family-in-law said when she did not conceive for nine years, she indicated the subtle pressure:

My sisters-in-law used to talk about it. My *atte* (mother-in-law) was indifferent. My sister-in-law said 'Every other family in our street has children. But in our house there are no children. If they were born in our house, we also could take them and stand at the front door.' Our grandfather also said the same thing. He used to say, 'I cannot see children in our house before my death' and 'I cannot touch them before I die. I got a child after his death.

8.7 Summary and Discussion: Cultural Schemas Identified

In the discussion about perceived reproductive and general health status and perceived etiology, cultural schemas (see Chapter 2) on health, illness and reproduction, which motivate the reproductive health behaviour of women, can clearly be identified. We elaborate on these cultural schemas and make a link with findings in Chapters 6 and 7, as well as with earlier research on pregnancy and delivery in the research area (Hutter, 1994).

By adopting a life course approach and thus situating child spacing behaviour in the reproductive career, we can identify

cultural schemas which are valid during different stages in the life course. By linking different events in the reproductive career, we observe that the schemas and beliefs behind reproductive health behaviour are part of a more or less stable and broader cultural meaning system. For example, the cultural schema of *hasi may* motivates behaviour relating to food and care after menarche, after delivery and an abortion. The cultural schema of pollution motivates segregation during menarche and menstruation and care in the first five days after delivery and abstinence from sexual relations. Most importantly, the cultural schema of heating motivates reproductive health behaviour and processes throughout the reproductive career: the use of oral pill and abortions; sexuality; menstruation and white discharge; pregnancy and delivery; post-partum amenorrhoea and infertility. The schemas of heating moreover relate to general health aspects such as the general weakness syndrome and to certain perceptions about the body (having no blood in the body).

8.7.1 *HASI MAY*

The concept of *hasi may* (tender body) or *aarishna may* (turmeric body) during menarche, after delivery and abortion indicates that women are considered to be vulnerable in particular periods. During *hasi may* or *arishina may*, women are assumed to be vulnerable, especially to evil spirits (*gaali*, *bhuta*) and the evil eye (*drishti*). Women need to be protected from these threats, which means that they have to stay indoors. During *hasi may* a woman or girl needs special food: sweets made out of wheat, milk and jaggery, fresh and hot food (no food leftovers), and soft food (instead of hard food). During menarche, these foods are to be given not only by the girl's family members, but also by the community and by distant family members who have a responsibility to provide food to the girl. The fact that women are seen as being vulnerable in these periods indicates that people are aware that these are crucial periods and events in which morbidity and mortality can be high. On asking women about their common health problems, women indeed mentioned *hasi may* to be a major health problem in the villages.

The cultural schema on *hasi may* including segregation, food

intake, and body care' motivates reproductive health behaviour of girls and women in these vulnerable periods. It is clear that the cultural schema motivates behaviour within social interaction (see D'Andrade, Chapter 2), female family members especially ensure proper behaviour at these times.

8.7.2 POLLUTION

When girls reach menarche, they are considered to be impure for five days, and are not allowed to touch anything, and they are given bath and food 'from a distance'. These five days of segregation are also observed after delivery; the pollution of birth is removed after five days (on *aidesi*). The schema of pollution motivates, at the time of menarche, segregation behaviour among almost all caste groups.

In addition, the period of menstruation is considered to be polluting, and women of higher caste are segregated (sit outside) for those five days. The schema thus motivates segregation only among a particular group of people. Adherence to a schema thus can be used to claim a certain social status. A Jain respondent, for example, who practises segregation every month, clearly does not approve of the behaviour of lower caste women who do not practice any segregation. Socio-economic circumstances determine whether women can adhere to the schema of pollution: quite a number of women of higher caste could not 'sit apart' during their monthly menstruation as there was no other person at home to take care of the cooking, etc. Economic or social factors thus can prevent schemas from actually motivating behaviour. The schema on pollution motivates worship behaviour among all the caste groups: none of the women conduct *puja* or light incense sticks during menstruation.

While in a state of impurity, either through menstruation or through sexual intercourse, one cannot 'approach the Gods'. Also sexual relations are considered to be polluting, as described in Chapter 6. The resultant schema of pollution prompts couples to observe abstinence during religious days or festivals or *pujas*. People firmly believe that harsh repercussions will befall those who do not observe abstinence during religious days (see Chapter 6).

8.7.3 HEATING

The concept of heating is embedded in the traditional medical system of Ayurveda[1] where food and other items are classified according to the effect they have on the body: heating versus cooling, light versus heavy, moist versus dry. The concepts of heating and cooling play a prominent role as well during pregnancy and delivery (see Hutter, 1994). The present research once again underlines the overall importance of the concept of heating. To understand this within the reproductive career more clearly, we summarize different findings, from the present research and former research both of which were conducted in the same research area (Hutter, 1994).

(a) Body Constitution and Processes in the Human Body Considered to be Heating

Heating Body Constitution: The body constitution of a person, i.e. the apportionment of the three humours, is determined at the time of conception. The basic composition cannot be changed, i.e. it remains the same throughout life (Lad, 1992: 18). Those who have relatively more *pita* are said to have a heating body constitution. In addition, each period in life is associated with a surplus of one of the three humours: adulthood is related to more *pita* (Lad, 1992: 20).

Heating Body Constitution Leads to Spontaneous Abortions: Earlier research (Hutter, 1994) revealed that women who have a heating body constitution more often experience spontaneous abortions. These women are advised to take a special potion, i.e. *beeven rasa* (neem juice) to cool the body down in order to prevent spontaneous abortions. Chapter 2 indicates a term for this in biomedical literature: women who frequently had spontaneous abortions are addressed as 'habitual aborters'.

Heating Body Constitution Leads to Irregular Menstruation: Some women attributed a hot body constition to be the cause of irregular periods.

Body Heats up After Menarche, Makes it Easier to Conceive: A

mother-in-law made an interesting observation, stating that girls who marry at a later age, that is more years after menarche, conceive easier as compared to girls who marry immediately after menarche, because 'their body has to be heated up'. So, a heated body makes conception easier. We could make a reference here to the literature on the biological model where periods after menarche are considered to be anovulatory for some time after the first menstruation (see Chapter 2).

Pregnancy is a Process of Heating: Pregnancy is perceived as a process of increasing the level of heat in the body: the foetus grows, some energy is generated and thus pregnancy is heating (see Hutter, 1994). This is quite a normal process. However, excess heat is considered to have negative effects (see later).

Less Heat in the Body: Weakness (no Blood, being Dried up): An Ayurvedic practitioner in one of the villages stated that general weakness, indicated by women as 'having no blood' and 'being dried up' indeed means that there is less blood in the body. And, according to him, there is less blood in the body because there is less heat in the body (see later).

(b) Heating Items Cause Illness Symptoms Related to Heating

In general, heating items lead to excess heat in the body and to symptoms such as skin problems, eye problems, a burning sensation during urination and headaches.

Oral Pill is Heating and Leads to a Warm Sensation in the Abdomen: One of the simplest—and rather innocent—effects of the heating qualities of the oral pill is a feeling of heat in the abdomen. The oral pill is also associated (see Chapter 7) with symptoms such as burning eyes, prickling sensation, pigmentation of the skin and so on.

Heating Food Leads to Pain in Legs and Hands (according to the Ayurvedic Doctor): Many women in the villages complain about pain in their hands and legs. The Ayurvedic physician explains

that these problems are due to taking too many heating items such as tea. Women could counteract this heating effect with cooling (*tampu*) but nutritious foods. However, as the practitioner says, women with pain in the legs and hands are more inclined to use allopathic medicines and injections, which in general are considered to have a heating effect.

(c) Taking Heating Items During Pregnancy Might Expel the Foetus

Heating Can Cause an Abortion (Either Spontaneous or Induced): The findings in an earlier research (Hutter, 1994) indicated that too much heat, i.e. heating food, work, sexual relations, allopathic medicines, alcohol, should be avoided during pregnancy as it is thought to cause abortions. It should be noted that pregnancy itself is seen as a process of increasing heat, and as such excess heating should be avoided. Instances of women using Anacin allopathic tablets (for headache) and experiencing spontaneous abortion are discussed in both the earlier and present research. Papaya is mentioned in both studies as having a heating effect and is used to induce an abortion.

Providing Heating Items Facilitates and Hastens Delivery: The earlier research also indicated that at the time of delivery heating items are provided to women to speed up and ease the birth of the child.

(d) After Delivery, when Women have Lost Blood, Heating or Energy-rich Food and Heating Conditions Restore Blood and Strength in the Body

Providing Heating/Energy-rich Food (after Delivery) Restores the Energy/Blood in the Body: After delivery, in the period of *hasi may*, women are thought to have lost a lot of blood and to be weak. The energy has to be restored by being 'heated up'. Hot water baths and charcoal fire (*benki*) are provided for a period of about three months. Heating up means that energy and blood are restored in the body. In addition, heating or energy-rich food (wheat, jaggery, hot rice) are to be provided.

In the period of *hasi may* during menarche, usually shorter than the period after delivery, the same energy-rich and heating food items are provided. The respondents do not really classify these items as heating, but more as energy-rich and nutritious. But the food items fulfil the same aim: to restore blood in the body and give strength.

Related to this, namely that blood has to be restored in the body by providing heating food and heating facilities, is the belief that:

When sufficient blood is restored, a woman gains strength, her menstruation will start again and postpartum amenorrhoea will end. In other words, the period of postpartum amenorrhoea will last longer when more time is needed to restore the blood. A frequent response was that a period of one or two years of postpartum amenorrhoea is quite normal.

(e) Heating and Menstruation

An Earlier Timing of Menstruation is Attributed to More Heating: Women indicated that when their menstruation was earlier than usual, it was because they ate something heating. They do not intentionally eat heating things in order to trigger menstruation. The interpreter, however, said that it is commonly known that eating *yellu* (sesame) and *kachu* (used in *pan*), or hard physical work will cause an early onset of menstruation. All these are considered to have heating qualities.

No Blood (Weakness) → Less Bleeding; Blood (Strength) → More Bleeding

Respondents said that when they are weak, namely when there is less blood in the body and they are dried up (*wana*), they have less bleeding during menstruation. Similarly, women felt that heavier bleeding during menstruation was a result of more blood in their body, that is they have strength. In general, heavy bleeding is considered to be good as impurities are removed from the body.

Here another link can be made: unless there is enough blood in the body after delivery, menstruation will not start and postpartum amenorrhoea will last longer. In Chapter 6, many

women indicated this relationship between delivery and post-partum amenorrhoea, namely whether there is 'blood in the body' which relates to more or less strength. Blood is restored in the body by taking heating and energy-rich food.

(f) The Oral Pill is Heating, Leads to More Bleeding During Menstruation, Causing Weakness and Inability to Conceive

Oral Pill is Heating and Leads to More (number of) Bleeding/ Menstruation: In the present research, the oral pill is regarded as having a heating effect and said to lead to more or a higher number of bleeding or menstruation. This means that women lose energy and strength.

Oral Pill is Heating, and one Becomes Like Dried Fish: In addition, by losing more blood, women lose energy and strength. The women illustrated such a weakness with concepts such as 'having no blood' and 'being dried up' (*wana*). One respondent described it as 'drying up like a fish'.

Women who are weak (no blood in the body) experience light bleeding during menstruation. According to another respondent, having no blood (due to heating effect of oral pill) also means that one is not able to conceive.

> When we take tablets, all our strength and blood will be lost due to the heat of the tablets. So conception becomes difficult.

Thus, because the pill is heating, it means more bleeding during menstruation which makes women weak and unable to conceive. By taking heating or energy-rich food, blood can be restored again, and menstruation will resume faster and the probability to conceive increases.

(g) White Discharge, Heating, Weakness

White discharge is thought to have several causes.

White Discharge is Due to Heating (Respondents + Ayurvedic Physician): First of all, white discharge is often said to be caused by heating, which can be counterbalanced by taking a cooling (*tampu*) home remedy comprising white hibiscus. Also the

Ayurvedic practitioner said that women who have white discharge should drink less tea and more milk (cooling). Actually they should take food that is cooling (*tampu*). What can also be taken, according to him, against the heat is *akki katchu* (water after washing the rice) and *jiirge* (cummin) and sugar. These items are also cooling (*tampu*). Nowadays, women resort to allopathic medicines (which are generally considered to have heating qualities).

White Discharge is Due to Sexual Contacts (Which are Heating): White discharge is due to sexual contacts with men who drink alcohol and smoke (which is considered to be extremely heating).

The respondents also indicated that white discharge is a consequence of sexual relations, which is considered to have heating qualities. Having sexual relations with men who additionally smoke or drink, creates even more heat in the body of the woman.

White Discharge is Due to Weakness = Less Blood in Body (Respondents + Ayurvedic Doctor)

White discharge is also said to be due to weakness and having less blood in the body.

There thus is a clear relationship, made by women themselves, involving heating, losing blood (due to an abortion, delivery or menstruation), the consequent weakness of 'not having blood in the body', possible inability to conceive, and white discharge. The weakness syndrome seems to be widespread. In the earlier research (1994), more than 60 per cent of women indeed turned out to be malnourished (Chronically Energy Deficient).

NOTE

1. We do not at all pretend to be able to give an overview of the elaborate health system of Ayurveda, but will only focus on those aspects as mentioned by the respondents, and remarks of an Ayurvedic practitioner living in one of the villages. It is clear that ideas from Ayurveda are mixed with local medical notions. For more information on Ayurveda, please refer to Lad (1992) and Frawley (1992).

9

Status of Women in the Reproductive Career

Chapter 7 on beliefs and perceptions about spacing methods and sterilization indicated that the major factors influencing spacing behaviour of women are attitudinal beliefs (discussed in Chapter 8) and normative beliefs. In other words, the majority of the women in the survey believe that their husband, mother-in-law and mother would not agree with them using spacing methods. The data indicate that women in the reproductive ages do not have much decision-making power themselves regarding the use or non-use of spacing methods and are strongly dependent on other people in their immediate environment.

In this chapter, we focus on the position of women, is as they are embedded in the socio-cultural context in which they live, in relation to important others. By adopting a life course approach, we study how the position and status of women in the reproductive ages have been given shape by social expectations and position in the preceding stages of the reproductive career, that is at the time of menarche and marriage.

Section 9.1 describes the status of women in the reproductive ages as based on data collected in the survey on educational level and occupation (see also Chapter 4), decision-making power and freedom to move. We subsequently look at the status and position of women at the preceding events of menarche and marriage. Reproductive life events are universal, they happen all over the world, in all societies, but are 'situated' within a context. For example, when these events are celebrated as rite de passage, as a transition from one stage to another stage, this is done in the way particular to and understandable within a society or culture. Sections 9.2 and 9.3 describe the transitions that took place for

women at the time of their menarche and marriage. We describe the ceremonies (rite de passage), the transitions taking place in status and social roles and social expectations for girls and young women. In addition, we describe the feelings of the women themselves about these major transitions in their life. Some information is provided as well about current customs and practices.

9.1 Status of Women in the Reproductive Ages

This section describes the status of women in the reproductive ages based on data collected through the survey. We first describe the socio-economic status of women, namely their educational status, occupation and earnings (Section 9.1.1). Also, information is provided on whether women can keep their own earnings and thus have some control of their own money. Subsequently, we describe the freedom of women to move within their own village, to another village, to their mother's place and to the market and cinema (Section 9.1.2). The decision-making power of women in matters such as market expenditures and health care of children is discussed in Section 9.1.3.

9.1.1 Education, Occupation, Earnings

Chapter 4 describes the characteristics of the survey population. To summarize, women in the survey are more likely to live in a joint family, as compared to the general population. The survey population is young: the youngest respondents (N = 7) are 15 years old, the eldest is 42 years old. Fifteen per cent are under age 20, while the majority are aged 20-29 years. The educational level is very low. A large majority (68 per cent) do not have any education at all. Only 3 per cent have completed secondary level, and 1 per cent have completed post-secondary education. When women who cannot read or write are included, the proportion of illiterate women is almost 80 per cent. On an average, the education of husbands of the respondents is somewhat higher.

Regarding their occupation, slightly more than half of the women are engaged outside the home, while one-fourth (24 per cent) are housewives, 32 per cent engaged in wage labour, and

24 per cent cultivate their own land. Just 7 per cent are engaged in salaried employment such as services, teaching and tailoring. Most women in the age group of 15-19 years are engaged in housework (38 per cent), while older women work more often outside the house. Of women who are engaged in salaried work (N = 491), 97 per cent earn cash. When the women were asked whether they could keep their own earnings, the majority (69 per cent) answered in the negative. A smaller percentage (9 per cent) said that they can keep part of their earnings, or now and then. Most of the women who could not keep their own earnings gave them to their husbands (73 per cent), their mothers-in-law (15 per cent), and fathers-in-law (2 per cent only). Age again plays an important role: older women (41 per cent) more often could keep their own earnings than younger women (4 per cent). Compared to illiterate women (20 per cent), more literate women (36 per cent) were able to keep their earnings. Also women in nuclear families often kept their own earnings. The factors of age, type of family and occupation are of course related to each other.

9.1.2 FREEDOM TO MOVE

Respondents were asked whether they could move alone in their own village, to the next village, to their birthplace, to the market and the cinema. Of all respondents, 25 per cent reported that they can never move alone in their own village. Of all women who were allowed to move alone (75 per cent), just 22 per cent had the freedom to do this without asking anyone's permission. The majority (62 per cent) always had to ask for permission to do so. The majority (53 per cent) had to ask permission from their husbands, 15 per cent from their mothers-in-law and 23 per cent from both their husbands and in-laws. The percentage of women who had to ask permission from their father-in-law, only 1 per cent, is remarkably low.

While 25 per cent of the women do not move alone in the village, the percentage of respondents not going alone to the next village is much higher: 78 per cent. However, almost half of the women travel alone to their parents' place. Familiarity of the place is perhaps the main reason for this. Among those who go

alone, the majority sought the permission of their husbands (73 per cent) or their husbands plus parents-in-law. Just 7 per cent said that they do not seek permission from anyone.

Majority of the women (65 per cent) said that they do not go to the market. This high percentage is not only an indication of lack of freedom to move around, and a subsequent lack of exposure to information in the marketplace, but also of low autonomy in buying one's own food. The remaining 35 per cent of the women stated that they went to the market, either alone (29 per cent), or with their husbands (30 per cent), neighbours, friends (22 per cent) or others. Only 3 per cent went with their mothers-in-law. The majority (73 per cent) of respondents who went to the market sought permission, especially from their husbands. A large majority of women (79 per cent) have no exposure to the cinema. Just 14 per cent of the women said that they go to the cinema with their family members; another 6 per cent stated that they went alone. The majority have to ask permission, either from the husband (53 per cent) or from the mother-in-law (21 per cent).

Analysing the related background characteristics, again age turns out to play an important role. Young women do not have much freedom to move alone in their own village: 40 per cent are not allowed to move alone in their own village; only 12 per cent could do so without asking any permission. This proportion increases drastically and consistently with increase in age. Among the older women aged 30 plus, 36 per cent reported that they moved alone without permission. A relatively lower proportion of illiterate women do not move alone in their own village (23 per cent, as compared to 33 per cent among literate women). More wage labourers than women who are engaged in cultivation and who own land could move alone without asking permission, suggesting a difference between women of different socio-economic status: poor women who have to engage in wage labour to survive cannot afford to stay at home, and have to move alone in the village.

Of the few women who go to the cinema, most are literate and engaged in salaried employment or other occupations, and women with better educated husbands.

9.1.3 DECISION-MAKING POWER AND EXPOSURE TO INFORMATION

Respondents were asked about their decision-making power regarding food items to be bought in the market, household expenditures, expenditures for festivals, health check-ups for children, their education and clothes.

Less than half of the women are involved in deciding about what food items would be bought in the marketplace (46 per cent), health check-ups of their children (44 per cent) and clothes to be bought for them (44 per cent). An even lower proportion of women are involved in decision-making regarding household expenditures (16 per cent) and expenditures for festivals (33 per cent). Women were relatively more involved (53 per cent) in decisions about the education of their children.

In general, it can be concluded that the decision-making power of women is not high and that husbands play an important role in all the decisions. Age appears to be important again: for all activities, decision-making power increases with age. Also, literate women have more decision-making power, except for decisions on household expenditures where comparatively illiterate women have more decision-making power. Also, women living in nuclear families are more involved in decision-making than women living in joint families.

Another indicator of status of women (see also Chapter 3) is the exposure to information, for instance group meetings such as those of the Mahila Mandals and information provided by radio and television. There is no active involvement of women in any group activity. About 5 per cent (N = 48) participate in the activities of the DWCRA (Development of Women and Child in Rural Areas) groups. Only 4 per cent (N = 37) of all respondents are members of a women's group, the Mahila Mandal. Only two women are members of a political party. The participation of women in group activities is higher among older age groups, although the total number was actually too low to make conclusions. In saving activities and Mahila Mandal activities, more literate women participate. Illiterate women participate more in the activities of the NGO India Development Service (IDS).

Less than half (48 per cent) of the women have a radio in the household, while the proportion of respondents with television amounts to 12 per cent. In the poorer hamlets of T. Ramachandra Nagar and Goutan Nagalavi none of the respondents own a television. The presence of a radio or television in the household is one thing. Whether women are allowed to turn it on and off, and thus have autonomy in access to information through these communication channels is another matter. Less than half of the women (43 per cent) said that they were allowed to turn on the radio or television, while the majority (57 per cent) answered in the negative.

9.2 Status of Women at the Time of Menarche

Given the low status and position of women in the reproductive ages, we determined whether we could understand this by looking at the status and social expectations of women earlier in their life course, i.e. at the time of menarche and marriage. In this section, we describe the status of the women at the event of first menstruation. We subsequently elaborate on the ceremony that was conducted at the time of menarche (Section 9.2.1), the experiences and feelings of women themselves (Section 9.2.2), and transitions that took place in social roles and socially expected behaviour after the event of menarche (Section 9.2.3).

9.2.1 Ceremony

As indicated in Chapter 8, at the time of menarche two ceremonies commonly are conducted. The *sannu soobhana* (the small *soobhana*) indicates the end of the five-day period of pollution when the house is cleaned. In families which can afford it, a second ceremony, the *dodda soobhana* (the big *soobhana*) is conducted. This is an important event indicating the transition of girls from one stage of life (before menarche) to another (after menarche). The second ceremony is conducted on a special day after the first ceremony. An auspicious day is selected, as determined by an astrologer or *pandit* who consults the *Panchanga* (astrological book, indicating auspicious days for different life events). The girl is again given a bath and made to

sit in a kind of *pandal* inside the house. Again, new bangles are given to her and the woman who has given her bath during the first five days. These new bangles should be green in colour.

A respondent described the typical procedures of the *dodda soobhana*:

> On the sixteenth day the girl goes to the temple. The *soodar maava* (maternal uncle) brings a *sari* and five types of fruit. He also brings flowers which the girl keeps in her hair. A bangle seller is called to the house on that day at around 11 O' clock. Then we have to go to a temple in the village, offer the fruits and coconut, *namaskara* (saluting) to God and come back home. Ali the invitees are offered lunch. After that there will be *dodda soobhana* and every thing is over.

Another respondent added:

> *Soodar maava* and other relatives come on the sixteenth day . . . they bring *sari*, garland to put on top of the head (*dandi*), fruit for *udi*, betel nuts and leaf, etc.

Several important aspects are included in the two instances just described. A *dandi* is a garland made of flowers prepared for special occasions such as the reproductive events of menarche, marriage, and the ceremony during the first pregnancy. The *soodar maava* (maternal uncle) plays an important role, as he does during other important reproductive events of his sister's daughter. Actually, a girl can marry her maternal uncle and many of the consanguineous marriages in the study population consist of these uncle-niece marriages (see Chapter 5). The *sari* given to and worn by the girl should also be green.

The *dodda soobhana* also includes the filling of the *udi* (*udi tumbuvudu*). The *udi* is the part of the *sari* that covers the front part of the woman's body, especially her lap. During a ceremony, the *udi* is the place where five fruits or grains are gathered. It can be filled with different kinds of grains and items (coconut, bananas, betel nuts, betel leaves, flowers, etc). During the *dodda soobhana* the contents for the *udi* should be given by the *sooder maava*.

After filling the *udi*, the girl who has reached menarche goes to the temple, often accompanied by other women. After visiting the temple and lighting the lamp, *soobhana* are sung which indicate the end of the ceremony. A typical *soobhana* song is:

Mellow in body, am a little woman
Well washed saree I ain't own
Wrapped in a saree, lent from the laundry:
The ceremony-pandal, ain't I stepping down.

Mellow in body, am a little woman
Well washed blouse, I ain't own
Wearing a blouse, lent from the laundry
The ceremony-pandal, ain't I stepping down.

Pour your fine sweet-wheat,
Palmful sugar sweet
Bring you the meal, come oh mother,
who bore the beautiful daughter
bless her with the meal she loves so dear.

Balls of wheat-flour-sweet
Bring along crisp-ghee-fragrant
Come oh mother, who bore
the beautiful daughter,
bless her with the meal she loves so dear.

Areca nuts palmful, smiling
white pan-leaves for chewing
bring oh mother who bore
the beautiful blooming daughter
blessing her.

(Translation: Arya)

After completion of the ceremony the girl can go outside again. In reality, however, girls are often kept at home for a longer period. The duration of staying at home depends on the socio-economic status of the household. On asking whether the ceremony has changed over the years, respondents answer affirmatively. The nature of the change, however, does not seem to be universal but to differ among the socio-economic classes. Respondents from the lower economic classes indicate that nowadays the ceremony is celebrated in a more elaborate way. A mother-in-law living in a more isolated village explained:

In the past the girl had to sit separately for five days. Some people from her mother's place (*tavaru mane*) used to come. But now it has become grander. Inviting people for food at the end of the ceremony is more common. More people are invited. There has been a lot of change now. . . . The customs

have increased. More people follow them. In our times for five days we had to sit apart. Then on one good day the *sooder maava* used to come and the *udi* was given to her. But it is celebrated now on a large scale.

The respondent seems to be indicating that in particular improved economic circumstances have prompted people to celebrate their daughter's menarche in a more elaborate way. However, the process could also be interpreted as a sign of adoption of the customs and practices of the higher castes, a process indicated by the concept of Sanskritisation as developed by Srinivas (1976). A Gouli mother-in-law practically said that her tribe had adopted the customs and practices of Hinduism:

No specific procedures were there. For five days the girl was segregated and then we gave her a bath after five days. We do the *aarati* to her. After menarche we don't do anything. Only the family members will be there. . . . Nowadays it is celebrated on quite a large scale. In the past it was not done. Our time is gone now. Nowadays they have all started to do like you (pointing at the interpreter who is a Brahmin).

A reverse trend, however, is that the ceremony of menarche is celebrated to a lesser extent, which seems to be the case especially among the higher socio-economic classes:

They don't do anything these days. In our time when a girl reached menarche, they would celebrate for 11 or 13 days. They would give her a bath early in the morning and before that they would apply *arishina* to her. *Kobri-kara* would be prepared. Relatives and neighbours would be invited and they would give food to that girl. But these days none of these is done. They say that the girl goes to school and therefore it doesn't look nice.

In the first instance, this seems to indicate that people are more concerned about possible negative effects for the girl, namely embarrassment. But it turns out to be related to economic factors, i.e. people prefer to save the money and spend it at the time of the marriage of the girl:

They say that there is no point in spending 4,000-5,000 rupees on such a event. They say that they can use that amount some other time in a more useful way. People have become clever in saving money now. . . . In those days people considered it a beautiful and an auspicious event. But now they think that there is no need to spend money on feeding all the invitees. We have to invite all the relatives and apart from food, etc., we have to give them some presents. The total expenditure has increased. So today nobody

celebrates such an event. In the past the people were ready to bring everything in double quantity instead of the routine quantity. Today nobody does that. If we compare both practices, both are good. Today money can be saved. But those days it was a beautiful function, a form of expressing their love towards the girl. Today's people question about showing love to the children in this way. We can use that money at the time of their marriage. These days the dowry system has become more common. So what they think is that that amount can be used for paying the dowry. So they don't want to spend 10,000-15,000 rupees on such a function.

9.2.2 EXPERIENCES

We posed the following questions to our respondents: at the time of your first menstruation, whom did you tell about it? What was told to you? Did you know about menarche before your first menstruation? In addition, we asked about their feelings and the feelings of their parents. The different topics are related to each other, and therefore sometimes difficult to keep separate, as the following case study indicates:

I felt very shy. We were not allowed to touch anything. I was doing something outside the house. When my sister came outside for some reason, I told her first. . . . Usually we hear about such things. Our neighbours and elder sisters used to talk about it. In this way we knew about it to some extent. . . . I felt shy when I reached menarche. How to tell to somebody in the house? . . . (I) felt sad (*bejaru*) . . . because the news would spread in the whole village.

Bejaru literally means feeling bored, but it also means sadness. The feeling of *bejaru* is used quite often, as will become evident in the subsequent sections.

Most of the respondents told either their mother or another female family member about their first bleeding. The event of the first menstruation is a public affair:

She (mother) called one of her friends, gave me a bath, told me to sit in a place and did *aarati*. Then she told the other people in the village.

Another respondents recounted:

The news spread in the house first. When my grandmother came to know about it, it became public news.

Also in a more indirect way, people in the village easily come to know about the fact that a girl has reached maturity:

(My mother) . . . came to know that I had reached menarche. She gave me a bath with hot water. When the neighbours had asked her why she was giving me a bath, she said that I had reached menarche.

What did the mothers or sisters or other female family members tell the respondents when they reached menarche? In general, most respondents say that they did not tell anything:

Nothing special.

and

What to tell?

Only a few respondents said that they were told how to use cloth during menstruation. Most respondents were told what to do during the first five days of menarche (see Chapter 8). Other respondents were told that from then onwards their life would change:

My mother told me that after menarche it was different in a girl's life.

and

(My mother said) . . . not to go or talk with men. It is the duty of the parents or especially the mother to give precautions to their daughters. They should tell her about men. It is all for her good only, for her well-being. They tell us to be careful because in future we have go to our husband's house. We will still be very young and not able to understand many things. So the mother has to give information about such things. And we have to obey them. If we don't, they beat us.

On asking women whether they knew about menstruation before they reached menarche, most women said they did not know about it:

How could I know?

and

No, I did not know anything. We were like monkeys. . . .

Some respondents indicated that they 'heard' something about it:

When we live in one house, naturally we come to know something about it,

when one reaches menarche. If there are elder sisters in the family they know about it.

The respondents also felt that it is not necessary to tell girls about menstruation before the first bleeding actually starts:

It is not necessary that somebody must give information about it.

One of the respondents who had a daughter around 11 to 12 years stated:

Even if I tell her now, she may not understand it. So it is not necessary to tell her now.

On asking the question 'How did you feel when you reached menarche' a very typical answer was:

What is there to feel?

and

What is there to feel? It is God given.

Some, however, did express their feelings:

I didn't feel comfortable with menstruation. It was better before. I felt it was dirty. I was not allowed to move around inside the house during that period. We were not supposed to talk against the elders. We had to obey the elders. We could go only to those places where they allowed us to. Otherwise, we had to remain at home.

and

What is there to feel? I did not know anything and I had to listen to my mother. She told me not to go anywhere. I obeyed what she and other elders told me as I did not know anything. I felt shy.

The two examples indicate the importance of 'obeying elders' and the fact that young girls do not seem to know anything. Following the elders' advice was for their own good:

What they tell us is good for us only. And we have to obey our elders. That will be good for us.

A few respondents had positive feelings about their first menstruation:

I felt happy.

and

I was happy. . . . So that I could get married. If we don't get married, that is also problematic.

This link between menarche and marriage also becomes clear in the feelings expressed by parents. A respondent said that her mother was happy when she reached menarche, linking the event to marriage:

My mother was happy and was thinking about looking for a good groom for me.

Mothers expressed happiness when their daughters reached menarche:

The mother cares more for the daughter when she reaches menarche. She loves her. She takes care of her in every respect. She gives good food to her.

And another mother, talking about the menarche of her daughter and the celebration said:

The parents do it with love. They feel happy. The event of a girl reaching menarche leads to happiness. The parents feel as happy as when they get a son.

A mother's love and care for her daughter who has reached menarche is also expressed in the *soobhana* sung during the ceremony, as illustrated by the example provided.

Another respondent, however, said that her parents felt it a burden to celebrate the ceremony:

She cried as it was an additional burden. They had to earn money for food. This was an additional burden to them. Those who are rich don't have any problems. They have the confidence of celebrating it in a beautiful way. What should poor people like us do? It is an additional expenditure for them.

And in addition to the feelings of love and care, expressed especially during the ceremony, the mother-in-law who first expressed her happiness also felt sad:

I didn't feel happy. Actually I cried then because she was very young and had already reached menarche. If she had not reached menarche so early, she could have gone to school for some more years. She was 12 years old. So I felt sad and cried. I cried. Then my daughter also started crying. I was sad because then I had to think of her marriage and send her to a different place. So I cried. You feel sad if you sent your daughter to another house. See how the God has made this system.

Quite a number of respondents talked about the ambivalent feelings of happiness and sadness of parents, thereby linking the two events of reaching menarche and marriage:

> Elders will be having both feelings. They feel happy as their daughter has reached menarche. At the same time they feel sad as they have to get her married, and moreover they have to be very careful after a girl reaches menarche. Because in the village people tease the girl if she does something extraordinary. So they have both the feelings.

A mother-in-law explains how parents consider a girl who has reached menarche to be a burden:

> They think that our daughter has reached menarche, now we have to look for a groom for her. A girl who has reached menarche means that she is sitting on the chest of the parents. Within six months or one year they search for a groom and get her married. She then goes to her husband's house.

Clearly, transitions in social roles and expectations take place after the event of menarche. We elaborate on them in the next section.

9.2.3 TRANSITIONS

After having reached maturity, many things change for girls. Two respondents nicely summarized a couple of changes in behaviour:

> They told me to stay at home and not to go outside, to work in the kitchen, not to go anywhere. . . . And even if we go outside for work, we should come home directly. I was also told not to look at others and not to stop on the road to talk to others.

and

> (My mother) . . . told me not to go outside, not to talk to others unnecessarily and not to keep smiling at others. I also did not go to anybody's house. Only till menarche can we go anywhere.

We proceed to describe the changes in clothes and in behaviour such as going outside, playing, talking to boys, and working.

(a) Change in Clothes

First of all, in general, after reaching menarche girls change their way of dressing, some start wearing a long skirt (*lanka*) and

blouse, the dress so typical for adolescent girls in the villages, and others start to wear *saris*. A Muslim respondent said that she did not change the type of dress after menarche, but continued wearing the *churidar* (*salwar kameez*) which is the typical dress for Muslim girls. Obviously it is not the girls themselves who decide to change their clothes, rather there is social pressure, e.g. indicated by words such as 'proper', from especially the parents:

I was wearing . . . frocks and skirts. I continued them for some time. But later my parents told me to wear *sari*, because they wanted to get me married.

The meaning and status ascribed to clothes, the *lanka* being considered as the appropriate clothing for young girls, the *sari* for women, is clearly indicted here.

Not all women complied with the expected change in clothing. A higher educated woman (SSLC) said that she refused to wear the clothes which others thought to be appropriate for her after reaching menarche:

I was wearing long skirt (*lanka*) and blouse. My grandmother always used to scold me. She was the only one who forced me to wear *sari*. Others didn't force me to wear it. I wore a long skirt till I got married, thereafter I started to wear *saris*. People were talking like anything, because I was wearing long skirts. But I didn't care about it, because I was not wrong in my behaviour.

(b) Not Going Outside or in the Dark

But more than the change in clothes, behavioural changes take place. Freedom to move around is restricted:

They do not send us out after menarche. We had to stay at home.

and

We always had to be home.

Certainly, outings in the evening are restricted:

There are rules. Usually we did not go outside. Even if we went, we had to return home before seven o'clock.

If a girl goes out she has to be accompanied by others:

Earlier I used to go out, but after menarche I was not allowed to go out. I was allowed to go with my mother and brother. They did not send me with others.

When asked what the respondents felt about this restriction of freedom to move around, a typical answer was they felt *bejaru* (bored or sad):

> Before menarche we used to move outside freely. But after menarche that was not possible. We had to be at home only. So, I felt bored/sad (*bejaru*). We friends used to go outside before menarche. But after menarche we were not allowed to go outside. I was not happy about that.

Of course, nowadays more girls do go to school. But the number of girls completing higher education such as up to SSLC (standard ten, i.e. when children are around 16 years) is still very low. Even while following higher education, girls are restricted in their freedom outside the house after having reached menarche. A respondent who did not have any problem in sending her daughter to school, said that there is a limit to the freedom:

> She should come directly home after the school hours. She should not go outside.

When the researcher and interpreter joked that her daughter could go to the cinema with her friends, the respondent said very firmly:

> No. I don't send her.

(c) Playing or Talking?

On asking women about the differences between the period after having reached menarche and childhood, i.e. the period before they reached menarche, the following responses were given:

> After menarche it was not like the small children. I don't go for playing after menarche.

and

> After menarche . . . how can we go to play? Everyone will scold us. . . .

Especially, playing with boys was no longer possible:

> My mother told me not to go out and play with boys like I used to earlier, because I had reached menarche and it would not look nice if I played with others. Then people start talking.

The strong influence of social control becomes very clear in

statements such as 'people start talking like anything' and 'everyone will scold us'.

In general, girls are warned not to meet boys or men, and to avoid eye contact if men visited their houses:

> They tell us all those things, not to go outside, not to look at men, not to be outside when men come into the house, etc.

While most respondents were allowed to play with girls, the following respondent could play only with girls who showed good behaviour:

> Even while playing with girls we had to be selective. They allowed us to play only with girls who were of good behaviour.

Poor respondents did not feel any difference between the period before and after menarche: they could not play even before they reached menarche:

> There was so much work to do that we got no time to go out for play.

However, nowadays some things seem to be changing, including more freedom to talk to boys. A mother-in-law said:

> about talking and playing with the boys . . . that is allowed. These days it has become more accepted. In the past it was not like that, we were not that free. Girls were not clever like the girls of today. If it was so earlier, it would not have been accepted.

But when we asked in more detail, it is clear that there are a lot of limitations:

> People are afraid. If a girl talks to a boy they enquire about everything. They don't allow the girl to do it again. There may be some people who think about what will happen if they talk to each other. But we don't allow it.

(d) Work

After having reached menarche, some respondents mentioned that they had to carry out more work in the house:

> They tell us to do all the household work.

and

> They tell us to learn cooking too . . . before menarche usually we do the washing of clothes, cleaning of vessels, bringing water etc.

Only a few were lucky, like respondent S, who said that she was exempted from any work in her house, even after menarche:

> They didn't allow me to do such work. They are economically better off and I was the youngest. So, I did not work much. I only did some household work.

(e) Reasons

On asking the respondents about the reasons for all these restrictions on girls who have reached menarche, the frequent answer was that the elders said so and that they obeyed the elders:

> That is what the elders say.

and

> They tell us not to behave as we did in the days before menarche, to behave in a delicate manner, not go outside, etc. We also don't oppose what they say.

All precautions—not talking to boys, not going out, etc.—seem to be taken to protect the girl and the family name, all with a view to marry the girl:

> They say it doesn't lead to good results. The girl shouldn't play with boys.

and

> (My mother and sister) told me not to go outside with other men or strangers because that would not look nice. Then people start talking. We were young and could not understand anything. We were not expected to make mistakes. So we had to listen to our elders. I did not go outside.

As it is quite natural for young girls and boys to feel attracted to each other, we asked the respondent's opinion about girls who do talk to boys. The answers of the respondents are quite clear, this kind of behaviour is wrong:

> It is not correct. Girls whose behaviour is not good only do that.

and

> Some girls may be like that. If they want to get a bad name they behave like that. People will blame us if we behave in such a way. So it is in our hands to get a good name.

The last quotation indicates clearly that it is up to a girl to keep her good name, and thus the good name of the family. The same respondent talked about the social control of other people in the village, and the possibility of someone speaking about the behaviour of an unmarried girl:

> Even if we are good, the people don't keep quiet.

She adds that therefore it is better that girls get married soon after they reach menarche. People talk anyway and it is hard for an unmarried girl to keep her name 'pure':

> So, it is better if the girls get married very soon after menarche. They give only one or two years' gap. Even though we want to lead a good life, people don't allow it. They should get their daughters married two to four years after menarche. When does a human brain keep quiet? If the marriage is late, then people start saying that she has not found the proper groom or the parents are not trying for marriage. That is why a girl gets married one or two years after menarche.

On asking the respondents what their feelings were about the fact that they had to change their behaviour after reaching menarche, respondents mentioned their feelings about marriage:

> It is a problem, of course. Moreover I had lost my mother and felt the loss more after reaching menarche. Elders' plans for my marriage also made me sad. People would be talking about it. So I knew that they were eager to get me married.

and

> Fear is natural. I was also very young. . . .

(f) Menarche and Education

The survey already indicated a low educational level of the women. Only 3 per cent completed secondary education (tenth standard, up to 16 years). Only this small percentage of women thus attended school when they reached menarche. One of them had to stop her education when she reached menarche. The reasons were that she had to travel quite some distance, alone, and after having reached menarche this was not allowed. Two other respondents continued their education after having reached menarche. The other higher educated respondent, who had

finished standard 10, tells about the conflicts between her grandmother, her father and her regarding the continuation of her education after she reached menarche. When she reached menarche she was taking her standard 9 exams:

> She (sister) advised me not to tell anybody else in the house, because they would stop me from going to school. She had to stop going to school when she reached menarche. So she told me to keep quiet. But my father was not like that. So I told the people in my house. Our grandmother was staying with us. She was of old ideology. She didn't want me to go to school after that. But my father didn't want me to stop education in the middle. So he said 'let her complete school education.' Anyway only one year was left by that time. So I continued going to school. My grandmother scolded me a lot. She scolded my father also. My father was not of the old type and sent me to school again.

We wanted to know whether the women who went to school received more information about menstruation or talked about it more within the peer group of fellow students. While in the first instance one of the respondents said:

> Yes, there were many girls and we were talking about each other's experiences,

she added:

> We were not talking that openly. How can we?

On asking whether teachers provided information:

> No. A girl knows about it whenever she gets it.

(g) Link between Menarche and Marriage

Reaching maturity is clearly related to a girl being ready to get married. The survey indicates that of all 951 women, 14 per cent married before they reached menarche (see Chapter 5). Of those who married after reaching menarche, the majority (60 per cent) wedded between the ages of 13 and 16 years. The average duration between menarche and marriage for this group was 12.5 months. Overall, one year after menarche, two-thirds of all women had consummated their marriage. In an in-depth interview, a higher educated woman talked about the naturalness of proposals coming in after a girl reached menarche:

> It is natural that proposals come, whenever girls are of the age of menarche.

Respondents mostly obeyed their parents in their wish for a marriage:

> (my parents) . . . were talking about it even though I was not ready for marriage so soon. But they didn't listen. They wanted me to obey them and I got married.

Even if the parents are not in favour of an early marriage, elders sometimes decided about the proposal, as one respondent related:

> I had reached menarche. So my father had told them that they were not in a hurry to get me married off.

But:

> The family of my husband came to see me when my father was not at home. The elders in the village finalized my marriage.

On asking whether her father did not oppose the decision, she answered:

> The proposal was liked by the elders in the village. . . . They can't be opposed.

In particular, the girls of the tribal group of Gouli marry soon after menarche, as a mother-in-law described:

> After menarche they don't do anything. We get them married after menarche and they go to their husband's house.

A few respondents got married later:

> I got my first menstruation when I was 15 years old. Six years after that, i.e. at the age of 21 I got married. . . . They started talking about marriage 2 years after menarche. They didn't want to get me married that early. I was going to the tailoring class also. So, they waited for some more years.

Nowadays, the duration between menarche and marriage is longer, and the attitude more relaxed. Parents seem to wait longer, after their daughters reach menarche to marry them off:

> Earlier it was like that. They used to start to look for a groom as soon as she reached menarche. But now it is not like that. People allow their daughters to be healthy and strong. Only after that do they think of their daughter's marriage. . . . After menarche we want to wait for about five to six years.

Another mother-in-law elaborated on the period between

menarche and marriage, and compared the situation in the villages with that in the cities:

> Marriages take place these days usually two years after menarche. Unlike in the past, they don't fix the marriage of a girl before menarche. But they don't leave the girl without marriage for 20-30 years like in the cities. They get married usually at the age of 15 or 16.

9.3 Status of Women at the Time of Marriage

As described in the preceding section, after the event of first menstruation, the social status and socially expected roles of young girls change considerably. Girls should 'behave nicely': not go outside alone in the dark, not talk to boys, keep the good name of the family, etc. The changes in social status are related to the fact that after reaching their first menstruation girls are considered to be marriageable. In this section, we describe the status of women during the different stages surrounding the event of marriage. We describe how marriages of women are arranged and which criteria are applied (Section 9.3.1). The several wedding ceremonies, indicating the transition towards the next stage in the life course, i.e. married life, is described in Section 9.3.2. Section 9.3.3 deals with the consummation of marriage, and Section 9.3.4 with the transitions taking place in the social roles of women after marriage.

9.3.1 Arrangement of Marriages: Criteria Applied

The previous section described how the respondents' parents often considered their first menstruation to be the sign to start thinking or deciding about their marriage. In the case of boys—as men indicated in the interviews—parents come to realize that their son has reached marriageable age by observing different behavioural patterns: the boy starts answering back, visits houses of other women and chats with them, stares and passes comments on girls who cross their path. The male respondents also reported other reasons for deciding on a marriage, e.g. the absence of any female at home to cook as the mother was ill.

Almost all marriages of the respondents were arranged (see

Chapter 5). In this section, we describe how decisions are made regarding the marriages of women, the extent of involvement of the women themselves in the decision regarding their marriage. In addition, we describe which criteria are commonly applied in the decision to marry a daughter. In other words, what do parents look for when they get their daughter married? In particular we also look at what qualities in a woman are sought after when she is getting married. Finally, we describe the custom of paying dowry at the time of marriage.

(a) Arranged Marriages

Almost all the marriages of respondents were arranged by parents, family members or elders. For most respondents, it was the husband's family who came with the proposal of marriage. Very often a relative suggested the proposal:

> Another person from T had brought the proposal. He is also a relative; he is a cousin of my co-sister. . . .

and

> My *soodaratte* (father's sister) came with the proposal.

In rare cases, the husband himself came first:

> My husband himself came to see me the first. Then the elders came. After that my father-in-law came to see our house, etc. Then the elders came again and fixed the marriage.

The wedding is arranged by the family and not by the couple themselves. Women are hardly involved in decisions regarding their own marriage. But, as the interviews among men showed, men too are hardly involved: in almost all the cases the decision that the boy should get married was taken by others, such as the boy's parents, grandparents, elder brother, other relatives, landlord or the elders in the village.

The female respondents indicated that they were just obeying their parents. A respondent who got married within one year of reaching menarche said:

> I was very young and I didn't know anything about it. It is very common in the villages that the girl gets married early. So I too got married. I didn't

have information and also not the desire to get married. . . . The only thing I had to do was to obey my parents. When they told about my marriage, I had to agree. . . . I did not feel anything. I had to obey my parents, that is all.

Also, one male respondent indicated:

I did not see the girl before. . . . I did as I was told by my father and mother. . . .

Nowadays boys and girls are said to be more involved and to see each other at least once, usually during the ceremony of *hannu idudu*:

Today's practice is that the boy also comes to see the girl and her house. . . . The boy has to see the girl and the girl has to see the boy now. In the past only the parents used to see the girl and boy and fix the marriage.

Also more often the girl is asked whether she wants to marry this particular boy:

Yes. . . . We ask her. If she likes the boy she says yes.

But even if a girl is asked whether she agrees to marry a particular boy, she often relied on the opinion of her parents:

I had to serve water and tea when they came. At that time I saw him. . . . What was there to feel or to say? I could not say 'no' and I could not say 'yes'. Anyway a girl has to marry and go to her husband's house. So, it is better if we obey our elders. We have to accept the proposal they fix.

Also, as men indicated, if a boy attends the ceremony of *hannu idudu*, often he only sits and 'sees', he does not talk to the girl:

We sat like this (as we were sitting during the interview) and went back.

and

My role was nil. I just saw the girl, as you now see me.

A few respondents could play a more active role:

. . . then the boy is asked about his opinion. They ask the girl also, whether she likes the proposal or not. They fix the marriage only if both boy and girl express their acceptance. If the boy says yes, but the girl says no, then it is cancelled. The first thing is that the boy and girl should like each other. . . . I liked my husband and agreed to marry him.

A mother-in-law added that nowadays some things indeed might have changed, but other things remain very much the same:

Even now we consider family factors while fixing marriages. It is still common today in villages, but it is not like that in cities. They go away with the partner of their liking and come back and say that they got married in the registrar's office. But in villages the elders still play a role in fixing the marriage. The marriage is usually conducted in the temple or in front of the house. . . . They don't say that there is no need to ask the boy and the girl.

The observation that changes are minimal is also clear when we ask whether the couple can meet each other before marriage, and respondents react strongly:

No. We don't allow that. . . . We don't allow it. Suppose my daughter-in-law stays in the next lane here only. Until she is brought here to stay after marriage, we don't go there and they don't come here. If sometimes we invite them for a festival, then they come and go back again. We don't allow both of them to talk to each other, share a joke, etc. Going to a cinema as soon as the marriage is fixed is not allowed. If the boy and girl see each other today and accept each other, then the proposal is made the very next morning.

(b) Criteria applied

What criteria do parents and family members apply in accepting a proposal to marry their daughter? First, all marriages are conducted in the sub-caste to which people belong. Consanguineous marriages such as maternal uncle–niece marriages or cross-cousin marriages (see also Chapter 4 and 5) are also common. A major reason mentioned by the respondents for consanguineous marriages is 'to continue the relationship':

This proposal was within the relationship. So my parents gave importance to that point. . . . He is my father's maternal uncle's son. . . . They were of older ideas and they wanted to continue the relationship. If they had fixed my marriage somewhere else, this relationship would not have continued.

Sometimes at the time of marriage, a new bride often has to promise to give her future daughter for marriage within the family. At the moment of entering the house of the husband (described further on):

The husband's sisters hold our legs and ask for our daughter. . . . They hold the legs of the couple and ask for their daughter. . . . We have to get a daughter and give her to them. . . . We give them our promise.

The respondent tells that she has to keep that promise, i.e. to marry her daughter to her husband's sister's son (*sooderatte maga*).

Some respondents indicated that they would like to give their daughters to their mother's place, and to marry them to their own younger brothers (maternal uncle–niece marriage):

I have to give one daughter to my *tavaru mane*. Two daughters are not married into my *tavaru mane*.

Child marriages are still common in the research area. These marriages are often consanguineous and conducted at the time of other marriages in the family. Economic factor, i.e. saving money on arranging a separate wedding, is often the reason for marrying of more daughters or sons at a time:

(I got married) when I was 4-5 years old. (My husband was) . . . may be 10 years? My brother-in-law's marriage was fixed then. So to reduce the expenditure our marriage was also fixed. Ours is within the relationship. I am the granddaughter of this house. The marriages were being conducted for others, so they conducted our marriage as well.

In the interviews with men, two marriages were reported to be child marriages decided by grandparents who wanted to see their grandson married before they died. Almost all respondents are against child marriages on the grounds that such marriages are not stable. Often, as was said, the boys and girls thus married refuse to cohabit with their spouse once they grow up, as the couple turns out not to 'fit each other'.

Also important in deciding about a marriage are existing marital bonds between two villages. It is quite common for villages to exchange their daughters in marriage. Women are referred to as 'daughter of village X' or 'daughter-in-law of village Y'. In the research area, for example, frequent exchanges of young women have taken place between the villages of Veerapur and Mavinkoppa:

In the past some girls of my mother's place married and came here. So through them we came to know about this proposal.

Proposals are sometimes turned down as the village of the proposed husband is considered to be too far away from the bride's village. Obviously, as case studies indicate, the distance

between the mother's and husband's place should be short so that the woman can visit her maternal home frequently.

There were some proposals earlier. One of them was from as far away as Z. But they didn't consider it because it was a very far off place.

In Chapter 6, respondents indicated that it is nice if daughters come home after their marriage and visit their mother's house (*tavaru mane*).

Some parents decided that their daughters should be married to someone living in the same village:

My parents thought that both the sisters and brothers would stay in the same village, 'in front of their eyes'. So they fixed my marriage with a boy of this (husband's) family and did not consider earlier proposals. They wanted their daughters to stay on in the village and not go to a distant place.

However, the most important factors in accepting or not accepting a proposal are economic in character. Most respondents stress the economic situation of the future husband and his family. This does not mean the higher the economic status the better. The two families should be of a more or less equal status, i.e. they should match one another:

The elders preferred agriculturist. We are not educated. If the girl/boy is educated then the match should be according to that. We were doing household and farm work, so a farmer agriculturist is suitable for us. At their place we would have to work and earn. Here too, there is no change.

If the husband's family has a higher economic status, more dowry has to be paid:

The boy must be good. He must earn a good amount and must be capable of taking care of his wife and children or he must own a house and farm. Even if he doesn't own a house and a farm, at least he must be strong and capable of earning. Now we don't own a house or a farm. If a boy owns both these, there is a demand for cash or gold at the time of the marriage. From where can we get cash or gold?

In addition to the economic situation the merits of the family and the boy are considered to be important:

First they look at property. Then they consider the merits of the boy and the environment in his house. But first preference is given to property.

The interviews among men also indicated that economic criteria are most important. According to men, some families prefer a girl from a poor family, since she is expected to adjust easily with the family and not hesitate to work. Some others prefer a girl from a family of economic status equal to their own, so that adjustment is easier. The girl should be in a position to do all sorts of work, even carry cow-dung baskets. Thus, an agricultural family wants a girl from an agricultural background and not from a jobholder's family because the latter will not adjust to their family.

In addition, as the interviews among men showed, the girl's character is considered to be important. The elders accept only a girl of good character: she should listen to elders, should not answer back, should be ready to work in the fields as well as in the house, should be able to adjust to a joint or a nuclear family. The girl should not have a 'loose' character, i.e. should not have had any affair or relationship with other men. Not only is the character of the girl important, but also that of other family members including the mother and sisters. Elders in the bridegroom's family enquire about the character of the prospective bride with neighbours and other residents of the village.

Not much attention is paid, according to both women and men, to whether the couple like each other. Only a few respondents mentioned that the couple should like and complement each other. The respondents themselves sometimes looked at other things and had other expectations:

> I had felt that he must be *chanda* (handsome, beautiful) and have a good job.

One of the important criteria, however, to see whether a boy and a girl are suitable to each other is the match of their *saalavaali*, their names provided according to their horoscopes. Commonly, the *saalavaali* or names of the future bridegroom and bride are compared to each other. The names of the boy and girl (given to them at birth according to the planets) are compared on the basis of the astrological yearbook, the *Panchanga*. If a match is not found to be proper, there is still a solution: the name of the girl can be changed. She has to go through a naming ceremony before

the actual wedding and her new name should be printed on the wedding card.

(c) Qualities of an Ideal Bride

As already indicated, the character of the woman is important. What criteria should women live up to? A mother-in-law explained that there are differences in finding a match for a son and a daughter. While looking for a son-in-law, the economic status of the groom's family is important. While marrying a son—and thus receiving a daughter-in-law into the house, the behaviour of the future bride is considered to be very important:

> That family and their neighbours should be good. When we go to their house, we must get respect. This much we expect from the family to which either we give our daughter or from which we take a girl for our son. While fixing the daughter's marriage we consider the land and the house of the groom's family. If we fix the marriage of our son we take care about the behaviour about the girl, etc. We ask the neighbours what the behaviour of the girl is like. Everybody wants a good match. Sometimes even if they (girl/boy) are not good, when we ask the neighbours about them, they may say that they are good. In that case it is one's luck. But what we feel is, if we give our daughters to a good family, she can live happily. If we take daughters of a good family for our sons they also will be happy.

Other important qualities of a bride are her age:

> First of all they give importance to her age. They also find out information about the girl's merits, her behaviour, etc.

The interviews among men indicated that families with a son of marriageable age look for a girl of 'tender age'. The desire for a young bride is mainly in the hope that she will listen to elders, and will not have strong opinions of her own. She can be guided and moulded according to the traditions and manners of the bridegroom's family. An older girl, on the other hand, is supposed to have difficulties in getting adjusted to a new home. Older girls are also more likely to be interested in other men. Men also indicated that the difference in the age of the boy and the girl should not be too small (minimum two years) and not too large (maximum 10 years). The ideal age difference between spouses is thought to be five years. Maladjustment in marriage is more likely

if the age difference is too large (the boy is more than 10 years older than the girl).

Another respondent added:

> She should be intelligent. She should have studied up to the fifth or sixth standard or even up to tenth standard. These days the girl's family has to think of giving dowry and even gold . . . she should suit our house. She should be healthy enough to manage the household work of an agricultural family. She should be clever also. If not, at least she should have good behaviour.

During the ceremony of *hannu idudu,* literally 'giving the fruit', in which the marriage is fixed, the qualities of a girl are commonly appraised. During this ceremony, the family of the bridegroom-to-be comes to the house of the bride-to-be. Sometimes (nowadays more often) the bridegroom is present as well. The girl is 'appraised' in several ways. A male respondent recounted:

> We see whether the girl is *shudda* (pure) or not. The elderly lady who came with us took the girl inside and saw all. She asked the girl to remove her clothes and checked to see if everything was alright. If they like her, then they ask us : 'Do you like this girl?' to which we say, 'If you like her, then we like her too.

Some physical features, e.g. the feet and heels are checked:

> There will be five to six women. They take the girl into a room and check her. They do it when they come for *hannu idudu.*

and:

> They also check the back to see whether there are white patches.
> Some people don't like the girl's chest to be high. Some people check her feet, that they should be straight. They even check with a thread.

A mother-in-law explained this criterion of the thread in more detail:

> First the measurement of all the five fingers is taken. Then they take a thread three times that measurement. The girl has to stand and hold one end of the thread in her hand with the thumb. The total length of the thread should cross the level of *kumkuma* (or *bindi*) on her forehead. If it doesn't cross the *kumkuma*, it is not good.

If the thread does not come up to the *kumkuma*, the girl is not

believed to be able to be a good woman or *muttaide*, and the proposal is cancelled.

If it comes below the *kumkuma*, it is not acceptable. She cannot be *muttaide* for a longer time.

Muttaide literally means five pearls, indicating women who wear the five 'pearls' of nose-ring, earring, *kalu ungra* (toe-ring), *mangala sutra* (wedding symbol) and *kumkuma* (the *bindi* of red powder). The *mangala sutra* is the necklace, consisting of black beads and two golden pendants, and is worn only by married women. Also toe-rings, worn on the second toe, indicate the marital status of women. *Kumkuma* is the red powder used for religious purposes and often applied on the forehead. The concept of *muttaide* thus refers to women who are married and who are considered to be auspicious. *Muttaide,* five in number, are able to conduct ceremonies and offerings (*aarati*) on several occasions, including wedding ceremonies (see Section 9.3). However, there are degrees of being auspicious. A woman who is married, who lives with her husband and has children, is considered to be very auspicious. A widow can never be a *muttaide* and can never conduct ceremonies and offerings (she might even never be present). A married woman without children can be a *muttaide,* but she is less auspicious than a woman with children, though more auspicious than an unmarried woman. The concept of *muttaide* thus clearly encapsulates the status of women in Indian society, especially the importance of being married and having children.

Another respondent mentioned other physical criteria that a girl must meet. Teeth, eyes, and feet are looked at:

They check the eyes and teeth also. . . . For some women the left eye will be a little smaller than the right eye. That is believed to be good. . . . Even a squint is considered to be good omen. They tell the girl to stand up and check the feet. The full print of the foot should be seen on the floor. There should not be any gap. If there is gap, it is called *kuduregalu* (horse's leg). That is not considered good. It is believed that the girl with such feet doesn't stay at home.

A mother-in-law said that a girl should be beautiful. On asking what is considered to be beautiful, she answered:

If the facial features are sharp, we say that she is beautiful.

d

Being very fat is not beautiful. They must be of medium weight, like the women in our house. That is good. Sometimes the girl will not be beautiful at all.

and

The lips should not be dark.

A fair complexion too is important, as some respondents indicated:

We prefer . . . her beauty and fair skin colour.

However, others indicate that complexion is not important. The same results were found in the interviews with men.

Commonly the lines in the palm of the hand are also considered:

They checked my hands, and the lines in my hands. For girls they also check the lines on the palm. There will be husband and wife lines on the palm. If they join one another it is good. If they don't join each other, then it is not good. Such a proposal is not considered. There will be lines of money also on the palm. It is called *dhana rekha* (*dhana* literally meaning cattle, *rekha* meaning lines).

Special attention goes to the lines indicating whether a woman will be able to bear children and the number of children:

They look at the lines on the palms and also the fingers and toes. They said that I have plenty of rice. That is all. My mother-in-law herself has seen the lines on my palms. That particular line is meant to be in the shape of a wheat grain. Then it is said that there will be plenty of food grains in the house.

The link between grain and fertility of a woman is seen in many other customs during the wedding procedures (see later sections). Besides the lines on the palm, the patterns of the fingerprints are looked at. They can have either the shape of a *shankha* (conch) or *chakra* (turning wheel). On asking whether these criteria—applied to girls—are applied to boys as well, a mother-in-law said:

No. There is no such method. Let him be like anything. He should be strong and hard working or he should have a job. What is there to check in boys?

(d) Dowry or Presents

Remarkably, many respondents said that no dowry (*dakshine*) was asked for at the time of marriage, but mo them said that 'something was given' to the husband's famil typical answer was:

> They had not asked. (They gave) . . . half a *tola* of gold, a watch and a pair of dresses.

The fact that the respondents said that no dowry was paid can be interpreted in several ways. First, it can be an indication of the poverty prevailing in the research area. Indeed, a reason to conduct a marriage within a consanguineous relationship is often because no dowry (or a low dowry) has to be paid. A respondent who had three sisters explains that her father was too poor to pay a dowry:

> Nothing was given. Actually it was decided to give half a *tola* of gold. But that also they didn't give.

Whether gold is given and how much is given can also depend on the economic status of the groom's family:

> These people (husband's family) did not have any land. So my parents gave less money. They gave Rs. 500 and a set of clothes.

But as one respondent said, if more dowry is paid, parents can be sure that their daughter will be treated better:

> If they give more gold to the girl, she will have a better life.

Another interpretation of the common answer by respondents that no dowry was paid might be that the bride herself is not involved in the negotiations: the amount of dowry is decided by the elders of both families. However, often people agreed only later—after an initial negative answer to the question whether dowry was paid (thereby giving a socially desirable answer)—that indeed some dowry was paid. For example, the family of the bridegroom whose wedding we attended also said in the beginning that they did not ask for a dowry. Later on it turned out that they did ask and receive 1.25 *tola* of gold and a set of clothes.

In general, the family of the bridegroom *does* ask for a dowry, as a respondent explained:

> Yes. They ask. Sometimes they ask a lot. They may ask for four *tolas* of gold and Rs. 4,000. The parents may say that they can't pay that amount, it would be feasible for them to give Rs. 2,000 and two *tolas* of gold. If they like the girl, they agree to reduced the amount. Otherwise they don't agree.

A mother-in-law said that, compared to the past, nowadays more dowry has to be paid:

> Nowadays a lot of money is spent on steel vessels and household articles. It has become a compulsory thing now. A marriage means household articles worth Rs. 10,000, dowry or Rs. 20,000 and five *tolas* of gold. In our time, the boy's family used to give some Rs. 80-100 to the girl. It was called *teravu*. It was given by the boy's family to the girl. Only then would the marriage take place.

The interviews among men indicated that the male respondents understand dowry as 'cash demanded and received by the in-laws during the wedding'. Twenty-eight of the thirty respondents said that they did not demand a dowry. However, nine respondents reported having received gold in the form of ornaments for the bride, the quantity ranging from 2 to 23 gm.

Instead of a dowry, the girl's family can take the responsibility to organize and pay for the wedding:

> There was no dowry. Our responsibility was to conduct the marriage. We had to give him one *tola* of gold and a set of clothes to him.

The Gouli do not have a dowry system but pay a bride price (*teravu*). Two older respondents (mothers-in-law) explained:

> The groom's party gives dowry. They give *teravu*.

In former times, the system of bride price existed in the whole area. Some of the mothers-in-law whom we interviewed were themselves married within this system (see Hutter et al., 2002).

Besides gold and money, the bride brings household utensils:

> They gave pots, steel tank, plates, cups, spoons etc. . . . To him (son-in-law) they gave a set of clothes, *pataga* (kind of turban) and a watch. They did all the things according to custom.

The household utensils consist of

> Plates, all types of containers, *shavigemane* (wooden instrument to make the *shavige*), etc.

and:

> They also give a bedding along with the household articles.

Besides gold, money and presents for the husband, what is given to the bride? Most of the presents consist of saris (presented during the different wedding ceremonies) and jewellery, among them the *mangala sutra* or *taali*—the chain of black beads and gold, the symbol that a woman is married. The costs for the *mangala sutra*, i.e. the two golden pendants, are to be shared by the two families. One respondent said that although jewellery was given to her as a bride, she could not wear them:

> They (parents) had given me earrings, but they (husband's family) took them away. They (in-laws) gave us gold because that gold will be in their house only.

9.3.2 WEDDING CEREMONIES

The actual wedding ceremony consists of several stages. Commonly,

- the first ceremony is *arishna dina*, a ceremony in which turmeric (*arishina*) is applied to the body of both the bride and bridegroom;
- the second is the actual conclusion of the marriage, *akki kalu*. It literally means the throwing of rice (*akki*) and grains (*kalu*). It is followed by
- *ashada karya*, a ceremony that has to be performed before a girl can be sent to her husband's house. There are
- several *neeru madudu* (washing the hands or feet) in both mother's and husband's house often followed by a visit to the family temple. In this area often the Yellamma temple in Soundati is visited.

Only after all these different ceremonies have been performed is an auspicious day chosen for the consummation of the marriage, when the girl goes to her husband's house (*sose bartaare* or *mane tumbuudu*). As one of the Gouli respondent described:

First, all the activities (should be done) like *neeru madudu*, going to different temples in different places and arranging special *pujas* at home are completed. After all such programmes are over, they can live like husband and wife.

In this section, we describe very briefly the different ceremonies. For more details, see Hutter et al. (2002). We focus on topics such as the overall importance of astrology, the important role of the maternal uncle (*sooder maava*) and the overall significance attached to fertility of women indicated by different symbols during the different wedding ceremonies.

For the wedding, an auspicious day is chosen according to the *Panchanga*. As the astrologer in Mugad explained to us, some Hindu months in the year are more auspicious to conclude a wedding than others. In addition to the most auspicious period, the most auspicious day and time of the day (*muhurta*) are determined.

(a) Arishina Dina or Suragineeru

Commonly, on the day or evening before the actual wedding ceremony of *akki kalu*, *arishina* (turmeric) is applied to the body of both the bride and bridegroom. They call it *arishina dina*, i.e. the day of *arishina*. If the wedding ceremony is conducted in the bridegroom's place, the bride-to-be arrives the evening before. She is accompanied by other relatives or neighbours but not by her own parents:

I had come with five to six people. Among them four to five women from our neighbourhood will be there. There will be 2-3 men also. The other people came on a tractor.

Her parents came only for the wedding:

On the next day, i.e. the wedding day my parents came with relatives and others.

A respondent whose wedding also took place in her husband's place describes the ceremony of *arishina* and *suragineeru* as follows:

One day earlier the bride's party goes to the groom's place. On that day they apply turmeric and give a head bath using milk and *ghee*. New bangles

> are worn by the girl. . . . They do *suragineeru*. They hold a thread around and give a bath. *Suragineeru* will be done five times. During the night they do it twice and once before the wedding. At that time they go and invite the people.

Suragineeru thus is the bath given to the couple, five times, each following the application of turmeric by several *muttaide* before the actual wedding ceremony of *akki kalu* takes place.

We can observe some similarities here with the ceremony at the time of menarche (see Chapter 8): at the time of first menstruation turmeric is applied to the body of a girl, and a bath is given using milk and ghee. At that time, a girl is considered to be in *arishina may*. We can interpret this as a symbol of cleansing: here the removing of old things before the actual marriage takes place, and a new stage of life is entered.

All women of the family present at the time of the wedding receive new green bangles. The similarity with the ceremonies during menarche and first pregnancy is obvious.

(b) Akki Kalu

The official conclusion of the marriage is the next day, and is called *akki kalu*. *Akki kalu* (literally rice and grains) is the mixture of rice, grains and *kumkuma* (red powder) that is showered on the couple as a blessing, right at the moment that the wedding is concluded.

The last *suragineeru* will usually be given on the morning of the wedding day, after which the bridegroom is taken to the village temple and dressed up for the wedding—new clothes, ornaments, and a tiara (*basinga*). The bride too is dressed up, in a new sari, jewellery and a *basinga*. The bridegroom comes to the wedding *pandal*. The bride has to be carried by her maternal uncle (*sooder maava*) to the *pandal*. The couple face each other, and a curtain is held between the two of them. Commonly the bride lowers her eyes and cries. She holds a filled *udi* in front of her. A priest recites *mantras* and at the designated moment (*muhurta*) the bridegroom and the bride exchange garlands, and the assembled guests throw *akki kalu* on the couple, showering them with blessings. The couple are married.

During the meal and feast afterwards, the married couple eat from the same plate. The bride and bridegroom are generally surrounded by friends and relatives who tease them constantly. The bridegroom is made to feed the bride and vice versa: and the whole process is watched carefully and made fun of.

Usually, after the wedding ceremony, the bride returns to her mother's place for some time. More ceremonies are to be conducted before she can really move to her husband's place.

(c) After the Wedding: Ashada Karya

After the actual wedding ceremony, another ritual called *ashada karya* is essential. Without it, a girl cannot be sent to her husband's house:

> Only after finishing the *ashada karya* can a bride be sent to her husband's house and called back to *tavaru mane*. Until *ashada* is done the bride cannot be send.

A respondent explained the ceremony:

> It is done during the wedding itself. The groom's party is given a separate house. I have to wear the new *sari* brought by them. In *tavaru mane* (mother's place) our *udi* is filled and then I have to go there (husband's place). Again there they fill the *udi* and send me back to my *tavaru mane*. That is *ashada karya*.

The custom on filling the *udi* (front part of the sari) with rice or grains has been explained earlier. *Ashada karya* is also referred to in the villages as *udi tumbudu* (filling the *udi*). At the time of the wedding ceremony, the bride's *udi* is filled with rice in her mother's place. Now, her *udi* is filled at the husband's place.

(d) After the Wedding: Neeru Maadudu and Going to the Temple

Another ceremony is *neeru maadudu*. It has been explained in different ways:

> Turmeric is applied to the hands and then they are washed. The husband and wife are then made to sit together and there is *soobhana*.

But sometimes *neeru maadudu* is also explained as the custom of washing the feet:

> The couple have to sit together. *Soobhana* is done and the feet are washed with water and turmeric. . . . The wife has to wash the feet of her husband.

The ceremony has to be conducted several times, in both the bridegroom's place and the bride's place. Some respondents said that it should be done for five days each in both places. Others said that they completed it in one day.

After *neeru maadudu* the bride again goes back to her house. Only after some time will she be brought to her husband's house for the consummation of the marriage.

During the various ceremonies, *soobhanas* are sung. As during menarche and the ceremony during the first pregnancy (*kubsa*), the *soobhana* for marriage includes a text related to the event itself, i.e. the wedding.

During all the ceremonies, several jokes are made. Insisting on the wife or husband mentioning the name of the spouse is a favourite 'joke', blowing puffed rice at the spouse is another.

Some respondents mentioned a stage between *neeru maadudu* and the consummation of the marriage, i.e. a visit to the family temple:

> After the couple visit their family god's place, consummation takes place.

In the research area often the temple of Yellama in Soundati is visited:

> They take the couple to the temple, *Yellamma gudda*, after the last *neeru madudu* which is done in husband's house. After that they take the bride to her husband's house. They look for an auspicious day and bring the bride.

After the visit to the temple, the couple are allowed to consummate their marriage. Sometimes, depending on the circumstances, a bride stays longer in her mother's place:

> No. After marriage I was left there only for three months. After three months they brought me here. They thought that I was very young. So they left me there for three months. Because of some customs which are to be followed, I stayed there only after the marriage. I was there only till (the festival of) *Naga Panchami*. Then they found out an auspicious day and brought me here.

Another respondent added:

> Sometimes the consummation takes place almost one year later.

The fact that respondents so often use phrases such as 'brought to' and 'sent to' indicates the low degree of freedom women themselves have to move: they are brought or sent by either their own family, husband or family-in-law.

The different ceremonies make clear that the wedding is indeed a transition in a woman's life course, but that some time is taken to make the transition easier. There are so many ceremonies that the couple have some time to get to know each other better. Only after the ceremonies are over is the marriage consummated. We discuss this event in the following section.

For men too, marriage is transition in their life course. A male respondent said:

> I left my friends after marriage. We were like monkeys those days. Now we behave differently as we have become adults. We think and lead life ourselves, we do not listen to anyone's word. We are involved in our work and home affairs.

9.3.3 Consummation of Marriage

The event of the daughter-in-law coming to her husband's house is an important event and it is known as *sose bartaare* (daughter-in-law is coming) or *mane tumbudu* (filling the house). It is also called *hosadagi* by women, meaning 'coming to a new place'. The actual consummation of marriage is called *hasige madudu* (literally: 'making the bed') or *prasta* (especially used by Brahmin and Panchal respondents).

When all the ceremonies are conducted, an auspicious day is found to send the girl to her husband's house. There are several rules regarding the time to send a bride to her husband's house. For example, according to the *Panchanga*, as the astrologer explained in great detail:

> The new bride can only be sent to her husband's house on the fourth, sixth, eighth to the sixteenth day after the ceremony of *akki kalu*. Any auspicious day within the first month is also good, but during the second month she cannot be sent. Thereafter she can be sent in the third, fifth, seventh, ninth or eleventh month.

When the bride prepares to go to her husband's house, food is prepared in her own village, the *udi* is filled, and some presents are given. Again the *sooder maava* plays an important role:

> When we came from my mother's place (*tavaru mane*), we had to go to five houses for *udi*. They prepared sweet food and sent it with us. They gave a *sari*.

Another respondent reported in detail:

> The food is prepared. The *sooder maava* has to give the food items, the items of *udi*, a sari and a blouse piece. Food grains are mixed and the food is prepared. Then *udi* is given in nine or eleven houses. . . . They apply *kumkuma* (red powder) on us and give us some rice, betel leaves and betel nut as *udi*. . . . Then they sent me here.

Also the bedding is brought from the girl's house:

> At the time when we came here to stay, they brought the bed.

After arriving in the village of her husband, the food that is prepared in the girl's village is distributed among households. This exchange of food between the two villages is repeated when the new bride goes back to her *tavaru mane* for the first time.

The bride will go to her husband's house together with some people of her *tavaru mane:*

> My cousins and aunts, had come along. All *muttaide* in the relationship came, yes, all *muttaide* came. *Chigavva*,[1] *sodaratte* (father's sister), friends, etc.

The relatives usually stay for one or two nights. One mother-in-law said clearly:

> They go on the very next day after consummation. Why would they stay for more days here?

When the bride and her relatives arrive in the village of the husband, first of all the temple has to be visited:

> When we came to the main entrance of the village, they sent the oil, etc., for the temple. We had to go directly to the temple, light the lamp there and then we went home.

Then, the bride enters her husband's house. Some respondents said that nothing special is done:

They take her inside . . . nothing special is done.

However, others talked about certain customs, e.g. keeping the *udi*—brought from *tavaru mane*—in a special place:

The *udi* given to the girl in her *tavaru mane* will be kept in the *pooja* room.

For, the prevention of the 'evil eye' falling on the girl when she enters her husband's house, the following is done:

Then we have to do *namaskara* to all elders and also to the husband. Then we have to remove the *udi*. To prevent the effect of (evil) eyes, they throw some rice or *rotti* on both sides of us.

Fixing nails on the threshold of the house is another custom:

When I came for the first time to stay here, the nail was fixed. The bride has to put her right foot on the threshold and the nail is fixed between the first toe and the second toe. There is . . . one nail fixed for every daughter-in-law. We are three daughters-in-law and there are three nails.

Nails are, however, not only fixed on the threshold for marriages, also for other reasons such as preventing evil spirits (*gaali*) from entering the house or witchcraft (*kankattu*). A respondent explained about this custom of fixing a nail at the time of entering the house:

Whenever some dispute arises she can say that I have entered this house by crossing the threshold. She can show her right in that house.

Another, related, custom before entering the house is to kick a small vessel filled with grain:

Rice or paddy is filled in a container and the bride has to touch it with her feet and make it fall and then she enters the house. Only with the right leg. . . . Then the nail is fixed on the threshold.

The contents of this container can actually consist of any grain, rice or *jowar* or wheat.

A Muslim respondent whose marriage was consummated on the very day of the wedding, talked about another custom to ward off the evil eye:

They prepare red water. With that water they free the girl from the evil eye. Then the bride is taken inside the house and has to sit on a mat. The sister-in-law washes her feet with milk.

She also described the prevalent custom of asking the future daughter for a marriage:

(The sister-in-law) . . . asks for our daughter.

Then, on the evening of the day that the bride arrives at her husband's house, the bed is prepared for the couple:

If the day is good, they do it on that day itself. Otherwise consummation takes place on another day. It has to be done . . . in the night *prasta* is arranged for. . . . The bed is given by the girl's family. They also bring flowers for decorating the room, and also fruits. Different types of food are prepared and kept in the room. They place the lamp and light it.

How much attention is paid to the consummation of marriage depends on the economic status of the household:

The arrangements depend on their financial condition. Those who have more money spend more on the arrangements. In my case, it was not that special, because both families didn't have much money. There was a separate room for us. Some fruit and milk were kept for us. The arrangements were very simple.

The next day, after the consummation has taken place, as a respondent described elaborately:

The mother or *soderatte* has to remove the bed and both the husband and wife are given a bath from a distance. They don't touch us and we also should not touch anything. . . . First they put some water on us and then they touch us and give us a bath. After that we can touch anything. Then, the bride has to give *udi* of coconut to five women.

Giving a bath from a distance was discussed also in the chapter on menarche, indicating the removal of pollution, due to sexual intercourse in this case. Also the house is cleaned:

The next morning everybody takes a head bath. The whole house is cleaned. *Pooja* is done.

Pooja is conducted:

The priest is invited and worshipped. He is also served food. Five *muttaide* are invited to do *aarati* for the couple.

The couple are given a special sweet:

They are served *shavige* (sweet wheat preparation).

When the respondents were asked how they felt during consummation of marriage, the answers illustrate that fear is a common feeling:

> I was very scared on the first day. The next day also I was scared. Then during a period of one month or so I got adjusted to it. I had fear for three to four days and I used to be silent.

And rightly she added:

> Everybody will have fear for the first time.

She also mentioned the role her husband played:

> I had to adjust and I had to be free from fear. My husband also helped to adjust.

A Muslim respondent said that in her community, the consummation of marriage is on the day of the wedding itself. There is not, as in other communities, some time between the actual wedding and consummation of marriage, leaving less time for the couple to get adjusted to each other.

In addition, the answers indicate that most women hardly knew anything about sexual relationships:

> I didn't see any movies. I didn't know anything. I came to know about it only after I came here. Before that I didn't know anything.

and

> I didn't know anything then. How could I have known anything then?

Another respondent, however, said that girls are told something. For example, they are advised not to oppose their husband:

> They will know something about it earlier. Elders will inform about it. They say that it will come to everybody's experience. They advise the girl not to oppose the husband. They leave the girl in the husband's house and go. The girl can do nothing but cry.

A key informant said that girls are told 'not to oppose' and 'to cooperate' with the husband:

> Usually many girls don't want to enter the room. They resist going inside or they start crying. In that case, the elderly woman who has come along with the girl tells her about it. Sometimes the sisters tell her. Usually the mother doesn't tell her anything, because generally they don't talk that closely with

the mother. Girls talk freely with their friends or aunts. They convince her about it. . . . They tell her not to oppose her husband when she enters the room. She shouldn't say 'no' to him. They can also tell only this. My sister had told me when I got married. She told me not to oppose him at all and to co-operate with him. In the villages not all girls know about it.

However, at present:

These days generally almost all girls know a lot. They will know everything when they listen to others. They need not be told about marriage. Today's girls are more forward. It was not like that in our time. Today's girls read many books and magazines and watch movies. So they will know everything. They are capable of telling about it to others. Even the girls in villages are very modern. Most of them go to schools. In the past, villagers didn't send their daughters to school. But nowadays everyone educates their daughters.

One of the respondents who said that she did not know anything about sex when she got married, thinks that younger people nowadays know much more about sex, even before they get married. They learn about sex especially through the cinema, she thinks (and as commonly thought):

Today's children know everything about such subjects also, through the cinema. They don't need any information from us. We didn't know anything about such topics, we only knew about working and earning. They say that she loved this person and she loved that person. They talk like this, so it means they must know about making love. We know about it as we are married.

After the consummation of the marriage, the newly-married women go back again to their *tavaru mane*:

They send her here back after 1 month or 15 days. She has to stay for more days in her husband's house and a few days in *tavaru mane*. Both of the husband and wife go together and come back.

Especially in the first year, newly-married women often go to their *tavaru mane*, and also for festivals:

Once or twice in a month I used to go. . . . They used to visit us often. Whenever somebody came, they used to take me with them and then send me back. These people also didn't say no whenever someone wanted to take me with them..

Whether newly-married women are 'sent to' or 'brought from'

depends not only on the agreement with the family-in-law, as one respondent indicated, but also on her own family:

> I wanted to go much earlier, but they didn't come to take me.

Another respondent said:

> During the first year I went often to *tavaru mane*. For every festival they have taken me there.

She added that later on, she did not go very often:

> Nowadays these people don't send me there often. After the birth of the first child it became less frequent. Till two or three years after marriage I used to go there very often. My parents-in-law later said they felt bored without their grandson. So they sent me very rarely to *tavaru mane* after the child's birth. Later we got separated and started to live independently. Then it was problematic for my husband if I wanted to go to my *tavaru mane* often.

Similarly, a mother-in-law explained:

> They go to *tavaru mane* until they have 2-3 children. Then they find it difficult to travel with the children. After that they don't go to the *tavaru mane* often.

9.3.4 TRANSITIONS AND FEELINGS

When respondents were asked to describe how they felt after marriage, the answers indicate fear and uncertainty about staying in their husband's place, especially during the first days and months:

> For the first time there was fear. I didn't know what to do or how to behave. I didn't know what they would say to any of my actions. I didn't know what to do and when to do. So the fear was there for the first five days.

and

> In the beginning we feel afraid. There will be a lot of differences. It will be a new house, and people will be new. We will not know about the work and the people in the *atte mane* (mother-in-law's place).

Answers of some respondents indicate that it is quite common (and understandable) to have these feelings during the first days:

> Like every other woman. . . .

and

> Of course I was scared.

The fact that some of the bride's family members stay with her for some days in her husband's place was comforting:

> If somebody accompanies us for five days it is alright. Otherwise it is difficult. My sister was there.

Usually, as also indicated above, there is some time for the new bride to adjust to her new situation, and often she does not have to do fieldwork in the first month:

> For one month I only had to do household work because I was a *hosamodalagitti* (new bride). After one month I started to go to the fields, give the food and later started to do some work also.

Sadness about leaving their maternal home was indicated by almost all respondents:

> It is difficult to leave a place where we grew up and go to a different place to stay. For every girl it is a problem.

Differences between their *tavaru mane* and *atte mane* are referred to:

> I was very sad. Life in one's *tavaru mane* is different from the life in one's husband's house. In the husband's house we will have some fear. But in the *tavaru mane* we are very free.

However, after some time, as respondents indicated, one adjusts:

> It took me one year to adjust. To understand every aspect of a new house is very difficult. There will be tension.

and

> There will be differences definitely. We need one or two years to adjust to our husband's house.

One respondent indicated that indeed it was difficult, but there is no choice, one has to go through it:

> We had come here, that means we must feel good. After marriage the parents cannot allow us to stay there. Somehow we have to adjust here slowly. Now I am fully adjusted. What can I say other than this?

Another respondent indicated that things changed somewhat when she got a son:

> But now after getting one son, slowly things have changed.

What are the differences between *tavaru mane* and *atte mane*, as perceived by the respondents? The respondents indicated differences in the work they have to do. While in *tavaru mane* they can leave work and are sometimes excused, in *atte mane* they have to work hard:

> In *tavaru mane* whether we work or not doesn't matter. Everything is excused there. But here is is not like that. If the daughter-in-law doesn't work, they complain and say that why does she sit without work? She talks to everyone and doesn't go to the fields. She doesn't take care of the household, work, etc. When they complain so, we feel sad. I felt it is better to live without marriage. Why should I face trouble after getting married?

and

> In *tavaru mane* we do the work freely. It may be cooking or just give and take. But in the husband's house we don't feel free. We have to ask them before doing any work, even before cooking. We have to ask them what to cook and when to cook. But in *tavaru mane* we need not ask anybody as to what to cook and when to cook. There we have freedom to do anything, to cook anything.

Besides less freedom to cook whatever they want, women also have less freedom to go outside and to express themselves in their *atte mane*:

> There (*tavaru mane*) others listen to us. That is a big difference between *tavaru mane* and *atte mane*.

and

> There will be a difference. Here (husband's house) we have to be open to them. We have to do only those things that they tell us to do. We have to go where we are told. We have to obey them.

and

> We have to ask them before going anywhere. In *tavaru mane* we don't ask anybody to go anywhere. But in our husband's house we have to ask.

The control exercised by the family-in-law becomes clear from these examples. But it is not only the family-in-law which expects

a certain behaviour of their new daughter-in-law. The girl's own parents tell her to obey her family-in-law, to respect them and to 'keep the good name', not only of her family-in-law but also of her own family:

> (mothers say). . . that she should behave in a very good way with all; she should carry on all the domestic work, she should not talk against the parents-in-law and other members of the family. . . . They say that she should follow her husband and she should not say anything against him. She should understand him clearly and completely.

> Even today my mother says to me that I should not oppose them even when there is great difficulty, even if they scold me and beat me. If you tolerate everything, God will make you happy, they say. I have to keep quiet even if he scolds or beats, because I don't want to bring a bad name to my parents. Let him do anything, I should keep quiet. Otherwise, people will start talking about us.

She separated from her husband for three years and stayed at her *tavaru mane*. After three years:

> My husband came there (*tavaru mane*) to take me back. My brother told him that he would not send me if he continued to drink. He asked where I should stay if I went there. But my brother also thought that I had to go back and stay with my husband. That is better. It looks nice only if the woman stays with her husband. So he sent me back.

In addition, on asking what mothers told their daughters about how to behave in their *atte mane*, the following answers were given:

> They tell us not to talk against the elders in our husband's family, to do all the work as told by others, to obey the elders. That is all. They tell us to be *chanda* (literally beautiful). . . . It means not to have dispute with others, to behave in a good way, to obey everybody, to do the work as told, to smile.

and

> She had told me that no matter what they say to me I have to tolerate it. I should not say anything against them. Even if they get angry at me for some reason or other, I have to keep quiet. I must behave well with them.

Another respondent said:

> She told me to bring a good name to *tavaru mane*, in the future too. 'Till now you have brought good name to us, obey them all, take all the responsibilities and behave in a good way'. . . .

and

The parents tell us not to behave there (in husband's house) as in *tavaru mane*. They tell us to obey them.

Most respondents expressed their feelings and indicated differences between *tavaru mane* and *atte mane*. However, there were some exceptions to this. Some respondents faced fewer problems:

If we change our lifestyle to the lifestyle here, that's all. There is nothing special.

But her situation was different as

My mother-in-law was not there. So, there was no problem.

A few said:

My mother-in-law was very good. She taught me everything. She told me how to do things, what to do and what not. If there were guests she would tell me to serve them food, etc. Then I got adjusted. . . . If somebody came to the house, we had to give them water for washing, we had to serve them food. She taught me to cook. I used to ask her before doing anything. In this way I got adjusted. . . . I had to give him (husband) water for washing immediately after he came home. Then I had to serve him food. If he wanted tea, I prepared it. Moreover I had to obey everybody in the house.

Would it be easier if a woman marries within a consanguineous marriage, and already knows her family-in-law? Indeed one respondent who married her *sooder maava* and thus left her mother's place for her grandparents' place (mother's parents) said:

No. I didn't feel like that . . . (strange) because I have been here before.

And another respondent who married within the relationship said:

The people are very good. There will be many cases where the in-laws trouble the daughter-in-law. But here there is nothing of that kind. My *sodaratte* is my mother-in-law, she is like my mother now. . . .

But another respondent specified:

I was not that new to this family. But even then I didn't go outside much. If there were some guests, I had to take care of them. But even then I had some fear in my mind. I used to have some hesitation.

9.4 SUMMARY AND DISCUSSION: LINKAGES IN THE REPRODUCTIVE CAREER

By adopting a life course approach and thus situating child spacing behaviour in the reproductive career, we can identify linkages and similarities between the different events in the reproductive life course. Links and similarities can clearly be identified such as the overall importance of astrology, the *soobhana* sung during all ceremonies, green sari and green bangles, the *udi* being filled, and the important role of the *sooder maava*. Several of these aspects indicate the importance of fertility to women. In addition, the status of women during the reproductive ages and the low decision-making power of women about their own fertility and spacing behaviour can be better understood by looking at how women are socialized from the event of menarche onwards.

9.4.1 PERCEIVED LINKAGES BETWEEN REPRODUCTIVE EVENTS: ASTROLOGY

The events of menarche, marriage and first childbirth are closely related to each other in the research area. As indicated, the event of first menstruation indicates that a girl is ready to get married and indeed most women were married within a year after they reached menarche. Then, it is expected that within a couple of years women bear children and then undergo sterilization. As seen in Chapter 5, more than 30 per cent of women in the age group 15-24 years have already been sterilized, indicating a very low reproductive span between marriage and sterilization.

The in-depth interviews indicate another linkage between reproductive events as perceived by the respondents. We present a case study in which the event of menarche (timing, place, circumstances) is related to the subsequent future marital and reproductive career of a girl.

When we were interviewing an astrologer, a woman came for consultation about her daughter who had just reached menarche. In the first instance, the mother seemed to be consulting the astrologer for an auspicious time for the ceremony. However, there was more. The astrologer asked the mother where, when

and how her daughter had her first menstruation. That was: in the house, on a Saturday in a particular *nakshatra* (two-week period, each period being related to the planets), and she was wearing red and white clothes. The astrologer took all these factors into account and consulted the *Panchanga*, the astrological yearbook. He provided the results to the mother and later explained them to us.

The fact that the girl was wearing red and white clothes was fine. Other things, however, especially the timing were not auspicious. Based on these 'facts', the girl would face difficulties in her life: she would become a widow at an early age, have more men than her husband, and she would not have any children. Note that these statements clearly indicate that a proper Indian woman is married, has a sexual relationship with her husband only and has children. The time that this girl had her first menstruation was not auspicious, and her future did not look very bright. The mother, however, took it all lightly. The astrologer explained that much could still be done about it: the bad effects could be countered. He indicated that the *udi* filled during the ceremony of menarche should contain wheat, it should be covered with a red cloth, a thread tied around it seven times, and it had to be taken to the temple. The bad effects of the time of the event would be compensated for in that way.

Another mother-in-law also mentioned that her daughter got her first menstruation at an inauspicious moment, which she compensated for by donating a large amount of grain to the temple:

> When I asked after my daughter reached menarche, I was told that the day was not good. Then I had to give a good quantity of wheat in a new container. I gave it to the priest.

The examples above, and earlier examples in this chapter and others, indicate the overall importance of astrology throughout the reproductive career. The *Panchanga*, the astrological book which is released annually is consulted for many events in the reproductive career: to match couples (based on their birth names as provided on the basis of the *Panchanga*), and to identify the proper timing for the conclusion of the wedding, other wedding ceremonies, the consummation of marriage and so on.

The astrologer indicated that the attention for astrology has increased during recent years, and related this to the idea that people feel they have an increasing control over their lives. In former times, people left it to the Gods:

> Among the people? Yes. It has increased. This tendency was present among people in the past also. But now it has increased. Then people used to transfer their whole responsibility to God. But people want to ask more these days, such as before they take up a task. . . . We say that it has increased seeing the increased number of people coming to us. . . . Some educated people don't believe this, but the uneducated people believe. The reason for the increase in their number is that they believe that we tell them something helpful or beneficial. One more thing is that they think that the knowledge about everything has increased generally and therefore they get more benefits by consulting the priest to about their activities. They think that we select a good day for them to do their work. . . . (in the past) . . . also people asked about such things. But now it has increased. In the past people were more superstitious.

His story seems to indicate three stages of development: a first stage in which people attribute events to fate, it is 'all up to God'; a second stage in which people consult an astrologer; and a third stage in which educated people no longer believe in astrology.

9.4.2 SYMBOLS OF FERTILITY IN THE REPRODUCTIVE CAREER

At different events in the reproductive career of women, similar symbols are present, including the green bangles and green saris, the filling of the *udi*, and the grains and fruit included in the ceremonies.

(a) Green Bangles and Green Sari

During the ceremony for menarche, a girl wears a green sari and green bangles. Green bangles are also given to the woman who has given her a bath—from a distance—during the first five days. Also during wedding ceremonies, green bangles are provided to all female members of the family. At the ceremony during the first pregnancy (*kubasa*), the woman wears a green sari and green bangles. The image of the goddess in the Dyamavva temples,

worshipped by women on Tuesdays and Fridays, wears a green sari and a series of green bangles. The colour green itself can be interpreted as representative of fertility. The link with the agricultural cycle becomes clear in the worship during *raashi pooja* (harvest *pooja*) where the harvest and agricultural instruments are worshipped—the water pump in the field is worshipped, draped in a green sari.

Viewing the colour green as a symbol of fertility is of course an interpretation. When we asked a respondent—an elderly *panchayat* member—whether this meaning should be given to the green bangles and the green sari, she answered that there is no such reasoning behind these customs. She repeated, what is commonly said: 'The customs have been practised by the elders for decades, and people continue to practise them'.

(b) Udi Tumbuvudu

During the ceremony for menarche, the *udi* of the girl is filled with different items such as bananas, betel nuts and so on. Part of it has to be provided by the *sooder maava*. The custom of filling the *udi* of women is practised during almost all ceremonies in the reproductive career. The *udi* being the front part of the sari, the part that covers the lap, can be interpreted as a symbol for the uterus. During important ceremonies, it has to be filled with fruits or grains, these being symbols of fertility. As one respondent explained:

> In *kubasa* . . . that woman's *udi* is filled. *Dandi* (made of flowers) is put on her head and she has to go to the temple. They give a sari. She has to wear that sari to the temple.

Also, during the name-giving ceremony of a child, an *udi* is filled and given to five *muttaide*.

One respondent told us that according to her all these *udis*, filled during different events in the reproductive career, are completely different, that is, they are filled with different grains and fruits:

> Giving *udi* in *kubasa* is completely different. Five types of fruits—coconut, lemon, *jajikayi* (fruit), *uttatti* (date), *atti* fruit, betel leaves and betel nut,

akki kalu flowers, *churumari* (puffed rice), etc., are put in the *udi*. *Dandi* is also put . . . (during menarche) two coconuts, betel leaves and betel nuts are given in the *udi* after menarche, along with *dandi*. During the naming ceremony . . . betel leaves and betel nut, *uttatti*, *akki kalu* are given in *udi*. *Udi* is put in five parts in front of the god and to five women. They have to touch and hold the tottila (cradle).

The *udi* being filled with grains, rice or fruit of course can be interpreted as a symbol of fertility, with the *udi* symbolizing the uterus. This link between *udi* and fertility becomes evident in the statement of a respondent who describes the *udi* during the *kubasa*:

Eleven types of fruits are brought . . . (for *udi*). . . . The pregnant woman should not eat those fruits. The other family members can eat them. The pregnant woman should not eat them because it is like eating one's own children.

In Chapter 8, we mentioned that the word for vagina is *udibayi*. The *udi* refers to the front part of the sari, but also to the lap; the word *bayi* means mouth. We interpreted the word *udibayi* as the mouth of the *udi*. On asking one of the respondents whether the word can be interpreted as such, she said:

No. That is different. We say the child's head has not came to the *udibayi*. That *udi* is different from this *udi* of *samsara*.

(c) Other Symbols of Fertility

Besides green bangles and the custom of filling the *udi* with grains and fruit, other symbols of fertility can be observed in the different wedding ceremonies. The custom of throwing *akki kalu* (rice and grains) during the actual conclusion of the wedding can be interpreted as a symbol of fertility. Also, the custom of the new bride entering the husband's house and kicking the vessel filled with rice or grains can be interpreted as a symbol of future prosperity in the house and fertility.

During *hannu iddudu,* when the family-in-law visits the bride's family and 'appraises' her, symbols of fertility and prosperity are looked into: the lines of the palm that indicate that there is 'plenty of rice', the *dhana rekha* (line of the cattle) indicating prosperity, and the 'wheat' line.

9.4.3 THE ROLE OF *SOODER MAAVA* AND OTHERS

During the ceremony for menarche, the *sooder maava* or maternal uncle plays an important role: he has to give the green sari and bring items for the *udi*. The *sooder maava* also plays an important role during other ceremonies: the wedding ceremony and the ceremony during the first pregnancy (*kubasa*). A maternal uncle can in fact marry his niece, i.e. his sister's daughter. In the research area, uncle—niece marriages are quite common. Such marriages are conducted, as respondents say, to 'keep the relationships'. While entering her husband's house for the first time, a newly-wed bride can be asked by her husband's sisters to promise one daughter to them for marriage. Many respondents seem to be quite eager to marry at least one daughter into their *tavaru mane*. Their daughters thus will live their married life in their grandmother's place.

A marriage is not a contract between two individuals, but a contract between two families. The boy and girl are hardly involved in arranging and deciding about the marriage, although some changes can be seen nowadays. Often a proposal for marriage is formulated by or through a family member or relative. Elders play an important role in deciding about a proposal. In a few cases, the elders have more say in the marriage than the bride's or groom's parents. During the different ceremonies, family members, often living in the same street, play an important role. During the event of menarche, the girl is given extra, energy-rich food not only by her own family but also by relatives and neighbours.

Besides the fact that marriages are meant to strengthen bonds between families, they are also considered to strengthen the bond between different villages. While looking into a proposal, the distance between the villages is considered. It should be easy for the daughter to travel between her husband's and her mother's houses. The bond established between villages through a marriage is indicated in the custom at the time of consummation of marriage. When the bride goes to her husband's house, she takes food from her *tavaru mane* to be distributed among different households in her husband's village. When returning for the first time to her *tavaru mane*, she brings food from her husband's place.

In several religious or caste groups, especially among the Goulis, girls are exchanged in marriage between families and villages.

9.4.4 CHANGING STATUS OF WOMEN OVER THE LIFE COURSE

The survey indicates that women in the reproductive ages are hardly educated, and almost 80 per cent of them are illiterate. Young women in the reproductive ages tend to live more often in joint households and work more often at home than older women. Young women have less freedom to move around and have to ask permission from either the husband or the family-in-law to go out. It is clear that with age, the decision-making power and autonomy of women increases.

Education plays a role—literate women have more decision-making power and have more access to information. However, there are only a few higher educated women in the research area. Women wage labourers are more free to move around than women who are engaged in the cultivation of their own land, and thus are relatively better off. This suggests that the freedom to go out alone is dependent on socio-economic status. In general, it can be concluded that the decision-making power of women in the reproductive ages is low and that—according to women—husbands play an important role in all types of decisions.

By adopting a life course approach, we subsequently looked at how the status of women in the reproductive ages has been given shape by status and decision-making power in the preceding stages of the reproductive career, i.e. at the time of menarche and marriage.

The event of menarche is the sign for parents to start thinking about marrying off their daughter. Although things seem to be changing nowadays and parents seem to wait longer to give their daughters in marriage, the link between the two events is still made. Several interviews indicate that after menarche, the girl is seen as a burden, literally 'she sits on the chest of the parents'. After menarche, the girl has to be very careful and 'keep the good name' of her family and her own self, in order to keep marriage chances (of herself and her sisters, if any) high.

After having reached menarche, our respondents' position changed enormously. They were not supposed to go outside, certainly not after dark, and had to learn to carry out household work. They were not allowed to talk to boys and men. Their clothing style changed into that of a young woman (long skirt or sari). Some of these things seem to be changing nowadays, but respondents are still very clear that unmarried girls who talk to boys are bad. It is socially unacceptable that boys and girls show signs of being attracted to each other, even if they are only having a conversation. Almost all respondents indicated that their position changed after having reached menarche: the most important thing to do was obey the elders who told them how to behave in a proper way. To keep the good name of the family is another important thing to do.

Women did not have much control about whom to marry. The same applies to men who were also hardly involved in choosing their brides. However, nowadays boys and girls are increasingly being asked for their consent. But even if their consent is asked for, as respondents indicated, they do not always feel able at that young age to make their own right judgement and they follow their parents' wishes. The statements such as 'it is our fate . . .' on questions on what kind of marriage is best, indicate that women do not really feel it is within their control.

The way in which girls are 'appraised' during the ceremony of *hannu idudu,* checking whether they can indeed read and write, checking their feet, chest, and so on, indicates a dependency on not only judgement by physical characteristics but also on such a judgement by others. Boys are not 'appraised' in any way for marriage.

The importance of being married is visible in the concept of *muttaide.* Married women, preferably with children, are most auspicious and conduct all kind of ceremonies and *puja.* Unmarried women and especially widowed or separated women are not auspicious.

After marriage, women 'come and go' from their husband's and mother's house. The way our respondents express it: 'they did not take me', 'they sent me', 'they did bring me', indicates the low power to decide themselves when to travel. It is decided either by their husbands and in-laws or by their parents, brothers or

family in her mother's place, whether a woman will travel or not.

A clear indication of the status of women is how women are told to adapt to their husband's house after marriage and especially what their mothers tell them to do. After marriage women have to

- adapt
- adjust
- tolerate
- obey
- not speak against elders
- cooperate
- smile
- be *chanda* (nice)
- keep the good name of their parents . . .

In the in-depth interviews, the question what a good woman looks like was also asked. A mother-in-law explained in this regard the concept of *pativrata*, i.e. the Indian concept of a good woman and wife:

> She should be sincere to her husband. She should lead her family in a good way.

Later on she described a good woman and wife to be as follows:

> She should take care of all her responsibilities in a proper manner. She should behave in a good way with all others. She should have good company. She should care for her husband, children and other members of the family. Even if she goes for a job, she is said to be good if she works in a good manner in her office as well as in her house. If she spends all her time and money on unnecessary things, doesn't come home on time, then how can one call her a good wife? If she complains all the time about the husband or her in-laws, she can't be good.

A bad wife is:

> If she doesn't stay with her husband and keeps company with another man and goes off with him, she is not a good wife.

The same mother-in-law reflects on the differences between the present and past:

> Who feels shy now? Nobody feels shy. In the past, we didn't see our husband's face directly. But now they don't care about others. They just sit

together and talk to each other. We did not sit in front of each other and look at each other's faces. But now they sit together for meals even during the wedding ceremony. Nowadays something is given to them to drink together. . . . Very rarely did we talk to each other except when nobody was around. But now it is just the opposite. . . . We used to feel very shy, but these days the girls don't feel shy at all. They observe all the things in the cinema and follow it. In our time there were no cinemas. I did not go in the bus, because our body touches some other person's body. I did not like it. So I used to walk to my *tavaru mane*.

A female respondent talked about the relationship with her husband:

For a woman her husband is her God. So she has to be with him (having sex) with a pure mind. That is good for her. She should love him with her heart . . . not say anything against her husband; she must obey him, serve him food, do all services for him.

The interviews among the men indicated that in their view a good woman should:

- be good looking
- always smiling
- not argue
- not quarrel with others
- be good at work, both in the field and at home
- get up early in the morning for work
- behave according to the custom of the house
- fear and respect the husband, love him, do things he desires
- not keep relation with any person other than her husband
- take care of her husband properly (in all respects: meals, *tiffin*, water, bed)
- take care of the husband when he comes from work (provide water for washing feet) and keep food ready early in the morning and send him for work.

In addition, women are considered bad by men, if found talking loudly and laughing loudly which attracts the attention of other men. Some also reported that women who do not give water to their husbands when they return home, who do not get up when a man enters the room, and who question their husbands are not respectful. A good woman, as men said, should behave in fear of all elders and men in the family and outside. Display of chastity

by covering the head with the *pallu* while walking on the road is also considered a sign of a good woman. Initiation of sex by women is also not considered to be proper, as interviews among both men and women indicate. As a respondent said only one in a hundred women has a desire to have sex, i.e. women born with a certain star in their horoscope.

In addition, men were asked what a good man should be like. It is remarkable that fewer criteria were mentioned for men than for women. While the reported qualities expected from a good woman related mainly to sexual chastity, modesty, being respectful to others, the qualities that characterize a good man relate mostly to his behaviour in financial dealings and altruism. Although having relationships with other women is considered to be bad, that alone is not sufficient to qualify him as bad. Taking money from someone and refusing to give it back or picking a quarrel while repaying is considered to be the most important feature of a bad man. Men who pick quarrels with others, who do not work hard and those who spend all their money on drinking are considered to be bad.

Given the socialization of women from the event of menarche onwards, as described in this chapter, it is not really surprising that women hardly have any decision-making power in their spacing behaviour. Also, the overall importance of fertility in society is evident. As respondents indicated, after having the first child, their status becomes better and with increasing age status improves. The relationship between status of women and fertility is thus two-sided: women with more status have more control over their own fertility and reproductive health behaviour. But also, women who have proven their fertility and have children have more status in society.

NOTE

1. *Chigavva* is either the younger sister of the mother or the wife of the younger brother of the father.

10

Translation into Health Intervention

Spandana: Research for Action

The results of the research, as described in the preceding chapters, are the basis for the formulation of a reproductive health intervention called Spandana implemented in different villages in Dharwad *taluka*. The intervention is a collaboration between PRC Dharwad, PRC Groningen, and the NGO the Family Planning Association of India (FPAI), Dharwad branch. Spandana was launched in March 2000, immediately following the release of the initial results of the research. Spandana is funded by the Bernard van Leer Foundation and partly by IDPAD (Indo-Dutch Programme on Alternatives in Development), both in The Hague. Spandana has been conducted subsequently in 17 villages (first phase) and 31 villages (second phase) in Dharwad *taluka*, including the villages where the research was conducted.

The objective of the present paper is to describe how the results of the research have been taken into account in the development of Spandana. That is, how the research provides evidence for the intervention. We first describe Spandana's philosophy and characteristics (Section 10.1) and then focus on the translation of the research results (Section 10.2). Following the educational matrix of McGuire (1985: Chapter 2), we make a distinction between the

- target groups focused upon
- topics included

*This chapter is based on several documents about Spandana, and co-authored with S.V. Morab, branch manager of FPAI Dharwad; S.V. Kulkarni, FPAI Dharwad; and Sujata Panigatti, campaign officer of Spandana.

- content of the messages
- materials developed
- pre-testing and sensitization
- change agents implementing the intervention

We limit our account to the first phase of Spandana which lasted from 2000 to 2003. The second phase of Spandana, ongoing from 2003 to 2006 and including aspects such as sustainability, scaling-up and rapid research methodology, is described elsewhere (see e.g. Hutter et al., 2003).

10.1 Philosophy and Characteristics of Spandana

The principle behind the formulation of the Spandana intervention is grounded in the idea that results of scientific research on reproductive health, especially in poor societies, should not only contribute to scientific knowledge and output (publications) but should also return in a tangible form to the people concerned in order to improve their reproductive health status.

Spandana's name reflects its philosophy. Spandana literally means pulsation, throbbing or vibration. In daily life it refers to the concept—especially in music—of 'relating and reacting to each other', 'empathy', 'tuning in' and 'interaction'. In our case, Spandana indicates the exchange of information and interaction among the different participants, with due respect for each other's background, objectives and belief systems: Indian and Dutch researchers, the NGO FPAI, local artists who made the materials and most important the people in the community.

Spandana is developed on the basis of earlier experiences with translation of research into action in the research area. An earlier research on nutrition and health status of women during pregnancy and after delivery (Hutter 1994) was also translated into educational materials (flashcards and puppet plays) and used in villages around Dharwad by the village health workers of the NGO India Development Service (IDS).

10.1.1 Bounded Rationality

The basic assumption of Spandana is that people in the villages are no 'empty vessels': they have their own knowledge and rational reasons—in the given circumstances—to act as they do.

The research presented in the earlier chapters makes this clear. For example, women show bounded rationality in their desire to have a particular number of children and a particular number of sons and daughters (Chapter 6). It would be too expensive to have many children as they have to be dressed, educated and fed. Sons are needed to continue the family line. To have two sons thus is better, in case one dies. A daughter is considered 'to look nice in the house' and is appreciated especially for emotional reasons. It would be too expensive to have too many daughters as dowries have to be paid at the time of their marriage. Women also show bounded rationality, reasoning that they have to work in order to survive and are already weak and malnourished (*wana*, dried up), so they cannot afford additional negative health effects of using spacing methods.

10.1.2 GOOD, HARMLESS AND HARMFUL PRACTICES

The basis of the intervention thus is the information derived from the existing behaviour of women, and the practices, perceptions and beliefs of the women and men. The objective of the evidence-based intervention Spandana then is:

1. *To Refer to and Reinforce Practices that are Good Rather Than Focus Only on What is Misguided*

For example, the research indicates that most women are well aware of the fact that it is better to space children. The average duration of birth intervals is 32 months, but almost 30 per cent of the intervals are shorter than 24 months. Postpartum amenonorrhoea plays an important role in determining the duration: the average duration is 9 months due to frequent and long breastfeeding. The use of spacing methods is extremely low: less than 10 per cent of the women ever used a temporary contraceptive method.

The average ideal duration of the first interval is 31 months, the ideal duration of consecutive birth intervals is 36 months (Chapter 6). Women are very much aware of the need of spacing, as they themselves say (Chapter 6): 'If we marry early, get children soon and too quickly, we are worn out and look twice our age.' A Kannada proverb even indicates that having children

at a very young age has negative health effects: 'For playing child troubling infant (*aduva makkalige kaduva kusu*).'

Women have their own idea about why they think it is better to have a longer birth interval. After marriage, it is good to get to know one's husband and family-in-law and to have some time to go out with the husband. After the birth of a child, it is best to have another child when the older child can play and eat 'with its own hand'. These findings imply that in general Spandana does not have to convince women that spacing is good. Spandana can refer to the perceptions of women themselves, 'as you know, spacing children is better, because . . .' and then the different reasons as pointed out by women themselves are given. Referring to existing knowledge is not only thought to be more respectful, but also to be more efficient, as Spandana can focus on those aspects which do need attention.

While women know it is better to space children, many of them (40 per cent) appear not to know how to achieve this desired birth interval. Those who have an idea have only very limited knowledge about how the different spacing methods actually work (Chapter 7), what the reproductive system looks like, and what the fertile period of a women is (Chapter 8).

Spandana thus refers to the existing knowledge of women themselves and articulates their own reasoning and perceptions. Then, honest and complete information on the different spacing methods is provided.

Another example is the custom of *hasi may* after delivery: women who have delivered are segregated for a couple of months from their family members to stay together with their child in a warm place, get warm baths, massages, and energy-rich food. One definitely does not want to change this custom as it has mainly positive health effects (see later).

2. *To Refer to and be Neutral about Practices which Might Indeed Deviate from the Biomedical Model, but which are not Harmful*

For example, during *hasi may* after delivery, women wear a head scarf in order to ward off wind and evil spirits (*gaali*). This

practice is not known in the biomedical model but does not do any harm, so it is not necessary to try to change this custom.

3. *To Refer to and Try to Change Practices which are Harmful, by Providing Information from the Biomedical Model*

For example, during *hasi may* after delivery, women are segregated and believed to be vulnerable to evil spirits. When health problems occur in this vulnerable period, the woman might not be allowed by her parents to go to the hospital—as revealed in an earlier research (Hutter, 1994)—as she might be attacked by these evil spirits on the way. The woman in question died on her way to the hospital. The message to be provided here is evident: whenever health problems occur during *hasi may*, ensure that the woman sees a health worker either in the village or in the hospital. The possible effect of evil spirits can be countered by known traditional methods (Chapter 9), for example by holding a small lemon (*nimbu*). Another custom is that women drink less water in this period, as water is supposed to dilute breastmilk. The reduced water intake is not good for the woman, especially when she delivers in the summer. So women are advised to drink more water in this vulnerable period.

The key message here is informed choice. Spandana aims to provide honest and scientific information to people in the community, so that they themselves—based on the information given—will be able to make their own choices and decisions.

10.1.3 ETIC AND EMIC EVIDENCE

Spandana thus is evidence-based. We make a distinction between etic and emic evidence following Pike's (1969, cited by Harris, 1975) distinction between the etic and emic perspective. The etic perspective, namely the perspective of the outsider, often consists of the researcher's theoretical framework or the biomedical model based on which we observe reality (deduction) and collect the needed data. Data from the NFHS for example and our own survey are mostly etic evidence: scientific information collected

on the basis of the research frameworks. The data on duration of birth intervals, postpartum amenorrhoea and breastfeeding, contraceptive use (Chapter 5), based on the model of Bongaarts and Potter (1983), are good examples of etic evidence.

Emic evidence is evidence collected about the insiders' point of view: the perceptions, beliefs and schemas of people themselves. The information thus collected, often through qualitative methods and analysed according to principles of grounded theory (Strauss and Corbin, 1997 and 1998), constitute local (inductive) theories. Information on the heating effects of the pill motivating spacing behaviour of women, and on postpartum amenorrhoea not being thought to be related to breastfeeding but to lack of blood in the body (Chapter 8) are good examples of emic evidence.

Spandana takes both etic and emic evidences as the bases for intervention. Interventions will be more effective in this way, as people are assumed to be more able to relate to and digest information which is based on their own way of thinking.

10.1.4 COMMUNITY AND DEMAND BASED

Starting with the existing behaviour of women, and perceptions, beliefs and cultural schemas of women and men themselves, Spandana is a community-based intervention. This focus on the community is related to and a consequence of the theoretical framework that we adopted in the research. Chapter 2 pointed out that we need to know the actual spacing behaviour of women, duration of birth intervals, fertility levels and actual use of contraceptives (Chapter 5). But also, if we want to know *why* women space (or do not space), we have to go down to the individual level (methodological individualism, Smith, 1989) and study people's behaviour, their perceptions and beliefs within the economic, social and cultural contexts in which they live. The theoretical framework of the research thus determines not only the level at which we collect our data, but also the level where points for intervention are identified. By studying spacing behaviour at the individual micro level, we try to understand and explain the behaviour at the aggregrate macro level (see social theory, Coleman 1990). Similarly, by identifying points for

intervention at the micro level, the ultimate objective is to observe results, for example changes in awareness and knowledge about reproductive health issues, at the aggregate macro level.

In addition to being evidence-based, Spandana is demand-based: the needs and demands of the community are taken as the starting point for the intervention. For example, after sessions on white discharge, women asked—given their problems—whether it would be possible to have a health check-up by a gynaecologist. Spandana now organizes gynaecological check-ups once a month, which are visited by many women from different villages. In the gynaecological check-ups, the number of infections actually turn out not to be as high as we expected on the basis of the research, where almost all women complained about white discharge. The gynaecologists involved relate the generally reported problems of white discharge mainly to weakness and malnutrition. In these check-ups, all women are given iron and calcium tablets. In cases of infection, women receive a prescription for medicines or—if needed—are referred to a hospital. During the gynaecological check-ups, women also started to consult about problems of infertility (see also Chapter 8). Infertility thus becomes a topic dealt with by Spandana, based on demand from the community.

10.2 Translation of Research into Intervention

Spandana started in March 2000, immediately after the release of the initial results of the research. The researchers from PRC Dharwad and PRC Groningen started to work with the NGO FPAI, Dharwad branch. In the first months of Spandana, several workshops were organized where the translation of the research into intervention was discussed. The discussions took place between the three collaborators, but also involved the participation of external experts such as medical doctors, gynaecologists, nutritionists, experts in educational training, NGO representatives, and representatives of the District Health Office from the Ministry of Health and Family Welfare in Dharwad.

In the first meeting, the research was presented as a basis for intervention while FPAI presented it's experiences in health educational activities. Issues discussed were: topics to include,

materials to be developed and used, content of the messages, and target groups to focus upon. All these issues are highly interrelated. In the following sections, we deal with these different aspects. The order in which they are presented, however, is for the readers' convenience, and not necessarily the order in which they were discussed.

10.2.1 TARGET GROUPS

It was clear in the very first meeting that our target group would be in the first instance women in the reproductive ages and their mothers-in-law, as the latter group turned out to be highly influential in the reproductive health behaviour of their daughters-in-law (Chapters 6 and 7). In addition, husbands were found to be highly influential regarding the reproductive health issues of their wives (Chapters 6 and 7), but in practice did not to have much knowledge about reproductive health issues (Chapters 6 and 8). It was therefore decided that men should be included in a later stage of the intervention. Men indicated that they had no knowledge about these issues, because the ANM only visited the women in the villages (Chapter 7). During the implementation phase, women in the community appealed to Spandana co-ordinators, after having received information about problems of white discharge and weakness: 'we know it by now, but please also tell our menfolk'.

Women thus wanted their menfolk to be informed as well and men thus became a target group, sooner than we first had scheduled and planned.

Similarly, adolescents were scheduled to be targeted in a later phase of Spandana. A few women asked Spandana to provide the information to their unmarried daughters, so they would have the knowledge before they would left the village for marriage. Adolescent boys and girls were thus also included in Spandana, in a later stage. In fact, this order, i.e. a first focus on women, then men and then adolescents, turned out to work well: parents already knew what Spandana was about and allowed their unmarried sons and daughters to receive the same information.

In addition, some topics and issues were thought to be more relevant for the general public (see later).

which they started painting specific charts, in collaboration with resource persons and researchers.

It was essential that villagers immediately and easily relate to and absorb the educational material. The flashcards and posters thus depict the local village circumstances: local houses, dresses, and village environment. See for example Figure 10.1 for the local setting. The two women on the right are clearly married: they wear the black and gold *mangala sutra* around their neck and toe rings on their second toe. They wear typical village saris and have a large *bindi* on their forehead. Also, Figure 10.4 depicts the local setting in the village: the sari worn by the woman, the kitchen with its pots and pans.

The accompanying scripts are formulated in local Kannada and include concepts such as *hasi may*, pollution, and heating (Chapter 8). The accompanying scripts revolve around stories about women and men living in a village, dealing with several reproductive health issues. Story telling is still a tradition highly valued in the villages. When a script for example talks about 'Kamalavva from Village X, who lost her sister due to problems of delivery . . .', women typically identify with their own experience and react 'that happened to my sister as well' or, 'it happened in this village', etc.

For each theme, a series of flashcards have been developed, each series consisting of about 10-15 cards with accompanying scripts.

In addition, a few posters have also been developed. For example, the findings about the desired number of sons and daughters (Chapter 5) are included in a poster (see Figure 10.6). The objective of the poster, entitled 'Sons and Daughters are Equal' is to create more public awareness about the value of daughters as expressed by women themselves in the research.

10.2.5 CONTENTS AND MATERIALS

In the scripts and series of flashcards, the practices and perceptions of women and men are compared to and complemented with information from the biomedical model. However, there is variation in this. Sometimes, the practices and perceptions are taken as the starting point for discussion on a certain topic,

BOX 10.1

PARTIAL REPRODUCTION OF CHART ON HEALTH STATUS OF WOMEN

During the research, women in the villages reported several common health problems—general weakness (*ashakti*, *wana*), no blood in the body and being dried up (anaemia), pain in their hands, legs, waist and back. Often they attribute these problems to heat (*kaavu*) in the body. They also associate the problems with the use of various family planning methods.

ANAEMIA

One of the most common health problems reported by women in the villages is general weakness. These are the common symptoms, as perceiv`ed by the respondents:

- *ashakti* or *wana*
- no blood in the body, being dried up (anaemia)
- pain in hands and legs
- waist pain
- pain in back

All these symptoms of weakness are in a way consequences of the low nutritional status and physical workload of women in the villages. Their diet is not adequate. Women get pregnant and deliver children at short intervals. Women also perform various tasks continuously, inside and outside the home, without sufficient rest. They take care of the children, work in the fields, work at home, do the cooking and the cleaning. All this contributes to a general weakness and poor physical health.
The women said that the general weakness is due to insufficient blood in the body, and related it to the different symptoms mentioned above. In the biomedical model, this condition is known as anaemia.
....followed by information from the biomedical model on what anaemia is, what the causes are, how it can be detected and what can be done to counter anaemia.

WHITE DISCHARGE

Another common problem which women identified was white discharge (*bili muttu*).
When is bili muttu a problem?
Women reported that the discharge could be of different colours. Odourless white (discharge) is normal. White discharge with odour is a problem as well as discharge that is yellow in colour, with or without odour. If discharge is curdy, that is also a problem. Also, one of the

symptoms can be itching. It is advisable that both wife and husband approach the doctor.
What are the perceived and medical reasons of bili muttu?
Women themselves perceive *bili muttu* to be a consequence of:

- The general weakness of women, often related to symptoms reported for general weakness (pain in legs and hands, etc). Related to the heavy workload of women.
- General weakness, more in relation to reproductive problems such as an operation, use of contraceptives.
- Sexual relationships.
- Heat (*kaavu*).

These perceptions of women match the biomedical explanations of white discharge, i.e. as caused by general weakness, anaemia, and infection through sexual contact.
How does one prevent/cure bili muttu?
A traditional herbal medicine to treat *bili muttu* consists of white hibiscus, fried in ghee. Other traditional or herbal medicines are also used to counter *bili muttu*: the leaves of *karikeh* are boiled in water, and the mixture is passed through a sieve and the water is drunk. Similarly touch-me-not leaves are also used. These traditional medicines do no harm.
If *bili muttu* is severe, it is harmful and one must consult a physician.
As prevention, hygiene is to be maintained. Cleaning of the genital area is essential. A good nutritional status, i.e. a balanced diet, is also important.

after which extra information from the biomedical model is provided. Other themes, however, start with information from the biomedical model and only then refer to the perceptions of people themselves. Other cards consist only of information from the biomedical model, but include local concepts and perceptions in the accompanying script. For example, the series on the reproductive system includes the concepts of *kuusina cheela*, *marg* and so forth (Chapter 8).

To summarize, three types of flashcards can be discerned:

1. Cards that emphasize the existing 'good' practices, the social and cultural contexts, and add information from the biomedical model. Often a comparison between existing practices and the biomedical model is made.

2. Cards that emphasize knowledge; for example, as women and men appear to have hardly any real knowledge about spacing methods (Chapter 7), complete information on these methods is provided, while perceived side-effects (Chapter 7) are discussed in one of the flashcards.
3. Cards and posters that adopt an advocacy perspective. These cards focus more on creating awareness, for example, on responsible husbandhood and fatherhood, the status of women, and changes in adolescence.

We provide some examples of all three types of flashcards.

1. A good example is the series of flashcards on *hasi may* during menarche. Following the findings of the research (Chapter 8), the series starts with a card depicting a girl who is playing with boys and girls. She is wearing the typical dress for a girl and her hair is made in two plaits.

The next card, included here (Figure 10.1), depicts her subsequently as a girl who has just reached menarche. The girl has to sit apart from her family for five days. In the corner of her room, one can see the utensils used for drinking and eating which she has to clean herself and keep apart. She is already wearing the *lanka*, the traditional long skirt for girls who have reached menarche. The setting is a room in a village house, with a lamp and a niche in the wall. The expression of the girl's face can be described as a bit shy, perhaps tinged with a bit of fear. Near the door, some older women stand and talk about the girl. This reflects what the respondents revealed about how their mothers immediately announced the event in the whole village.

The next card (Figure 10.2) shows 'giving the bath' by five women who are auspicious, the *muttaides* (Chapters 8 and 9). The women wear the symbols of married women, i.e. *muttaides*: the *mangala sutra*, toe rings, nose ring, earrings and *kumkumma* (the *bindi* of red powder). A *sari* is held up around the girl during her bath (Chapter 8).

The first three cards of this series on first menstruation are meant to relate to the existing behaviour and perceptions. During the sessions, it was remarkable how women responded to especially the second (here first, 10.1) card: 'o, poor girl . . .'.

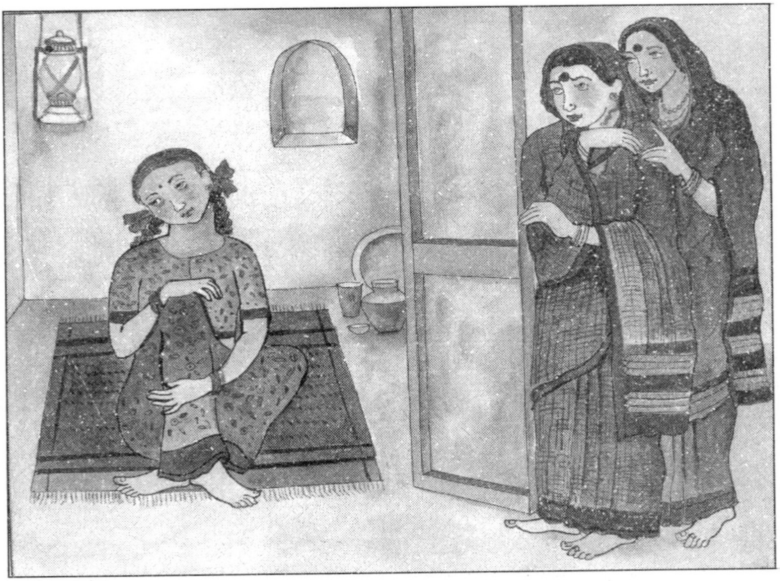

FIGURE 10.1: A GIRL SITTING APART DURING MENARCHE

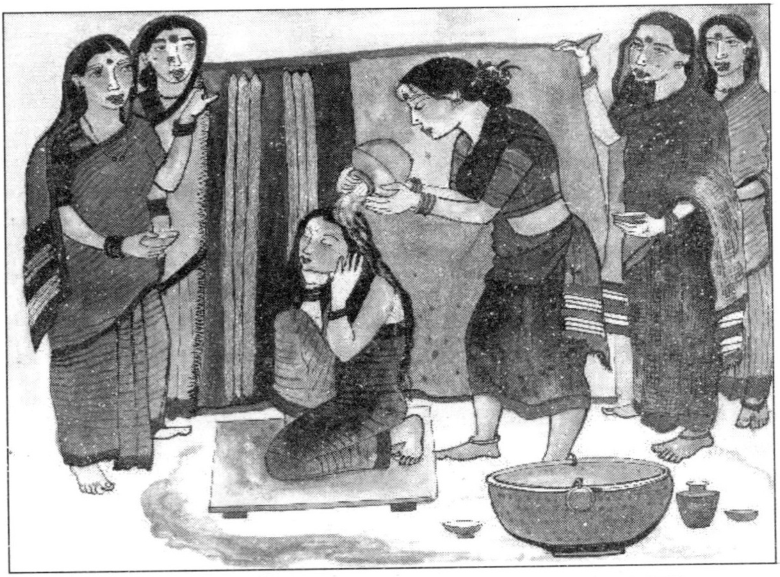

FIGURE 10.2: A GIRL DURING MENARCHE: HEAD BATH PROVIDED BY FIVE *MUTTAIDE*

Women immediately recognized the situation: this girl has reached maturity.

One of the following cards, then, combines the behaviour and perceptions of women themselves with information from the biomedical model (see Figure 10.3). The script of this card is as follows.

During the first menstruation the girl is in *hasi may* or *arishina may*. She is given extra food: sweets, energy-rich food, *kobri kara* . . . (seen on the left side). The food is provided so that she can get extra energy, regain lost blood and become strong. This is a very good custom. What you can think about is to add some other extra food, such as . . . (right side) green vegetables, eggs or meat (for non-vegetarians).

A similar approach was adopted in many other cards.

2. When there is lack of knowledge, for example on spacing methods, complete information is provided. The flashcards and scripts elaborate on all the different spacing methods: how they work, what the real side effects are, where they are available, when to take them, and so forth. In addition, during the educational sessions in the villages, all spacing methods are shown to the group. Figure 10.4 is a card from the series on the oral pill. The card provides information on the proper time to take the oral pill and where best to keep it. Like in other countries, women are advised to keep the pill in a place where it will not easily be forgotten so as to ensure daily intake. In the research area, it was advised to keep the supply of pills in the kitchen (women's space) in a metal trunk (to keep it dry). The best time advised is at night (indicated by a lighted bulb and the moon), after the evening meal (indicated by a clean kitchen). Note the village kitchen and the Indian crescent moon.

Then, the next card (Figure 10.5) refers to the negative side effects as mentioned by women themselves in the research. When the card is presented in sessions, both perceived and real side-effects of spacing methods are discussed.

3. Several series of cards and posters focus on advocacy and creating of awareness. For example, as indicated earlier, a poster has been produced to discuss the values of both sons and

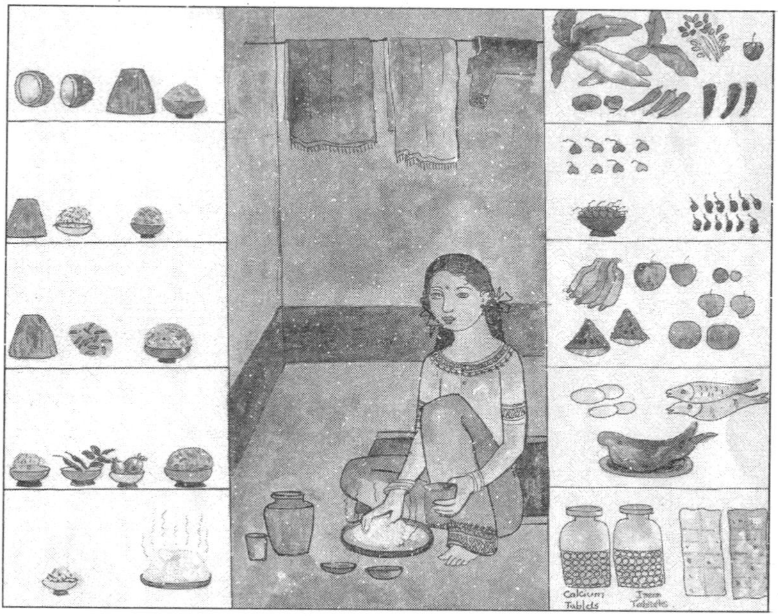

FIGURE 10.3: A GIRL DURING MENARCHE: EXTRA FOOD PROVIDED AND ADDITIONAL FOOD ADVICE

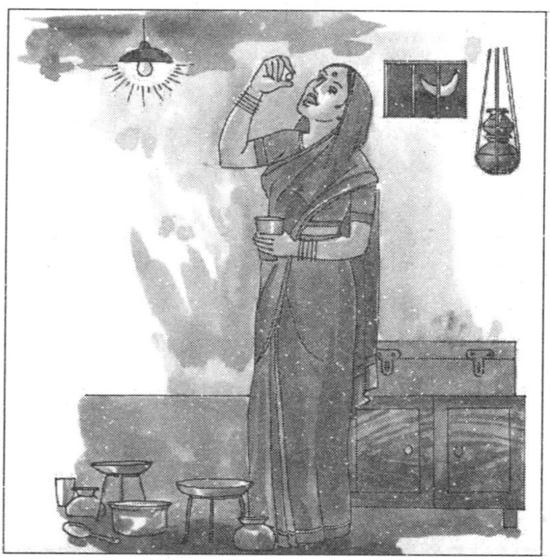

FIGURE 10.4: INFORMATION ABOUT ORAL PILL: WHEN TO TAKE AND WHERE TO KEEP

daughters (Chapter 6; see Figure 10.6). Actually, the poster is about the perceptions of women themselves, and no new information is added. On the left side of the poster, a son is seen working in the fields, continuing the family line (lighting the lamp), carrying the body of his parents to the funeral place. On the right side of the poster, one sees a daughter doing *puja*, a married daughter coming home with her children and the father obviously pleased to see her. Also, while on the left hand side, the son carries the body of one of his parents to the cremation ground, on the right hand side the daughter cries and decorates the body of her parent. Actually, the poster takes the perceptions of women themselves into the public domain with the objective of reinforcing existing perceptions about the values and the advantages of having daughters.

The different examples illustrated here might give the impression that the perceptions of the women and the biomedical model can be easily be combined and 'matched'. However, it is not that easy. The following discussion uses two examples to illustrate how difficult it sometimes is to combine the two. The issues taken up below generated numerous discussions among the members of the three organizations who were preparing the charts and the experts about the right procedure to follow.

For example, how was one to deal with the concept of heating so prevalent in the research area (Chapters 6 to 8). Matching the perceptions of women about heating to information in the biomedical model was possible in some cases. For example, the earlier research indicated that women should avoid heating items during pregnancy such as papaya, working in the sun, allopathic medicines, sexual relations, especially when their husbands drink alcohol and smoke. Actually, some of the items are not so different from what the biomedical model advises pregnant women: to be careful with medicines, alcohol, smoking. Similarly, the concept of heating as related to the weakness syndrome (being dried up, having no blood, having heat in the body) could easily be described in the biomedical model as being weak, anaemic and having a poor nutritional status.

However, the research also indicates that respondents think that the oral pill is heating. A long discussion took place during the preparation of the intervention, focusing on

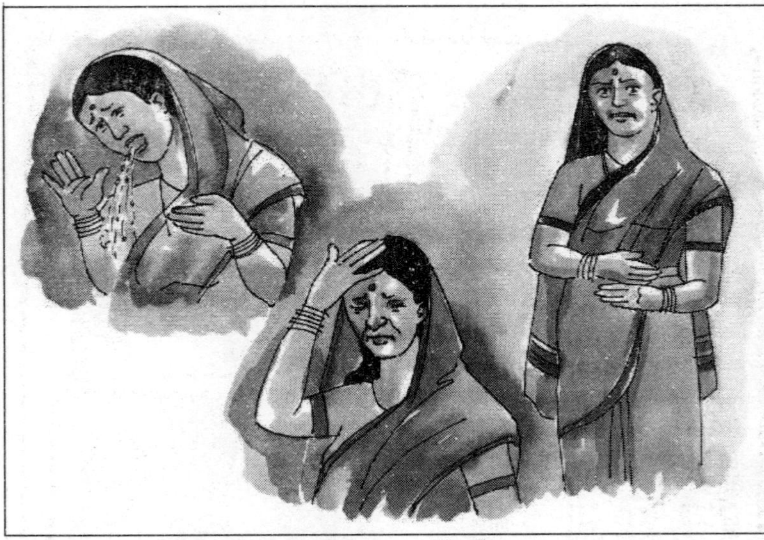

FIGURE 10.5: INFORMATION ABOUT ORAL PILL: DISCUSSION ON PERCEIVED AND REAL SIDE-EFFECTS

- Is the pill indeed heating? Depending on our own belief system or cultural schemas, some people agreed and some did not. Note that Indians were among those who did not adhere to the cultural schema that the oral pill is heating.
- Do we want to confirm the belief that the oral pill is heating? Or do we deny it? Is it harmful to believe that the oral pill is heating?
- And finally, how do we go about it in the intervention?

A solution found for this particular problem is described in the following sentence, included in the chart:

The oral pill is actually not heating, but if you do believe that it is heating, you can counteract the heating effects by taking cooling (*tampu*) items such as milk, buttermilk, or banana.

To cite another example, during our material preparations period, the Family Welfare Programme of the Government of India (GOI) did not encourage the use of the oral pill among women who were just married and who did not have a child yet. A very general belief (Chapter 7) is that the oral pill may lead to problems of conception. The FPAI followed the guidelines and

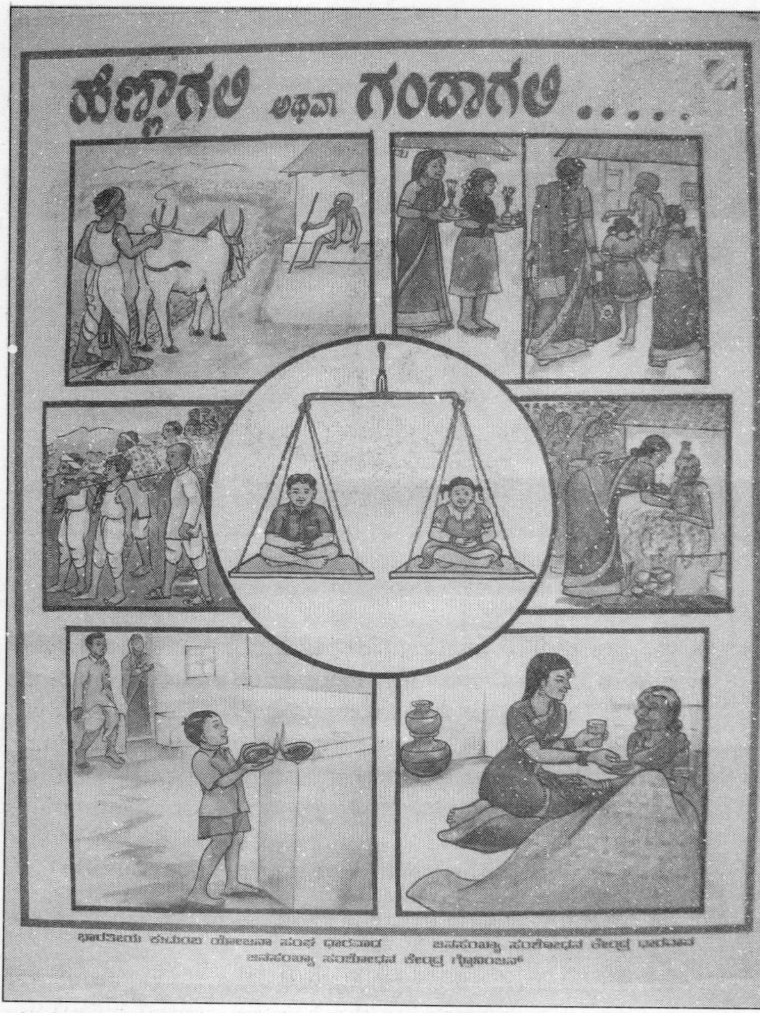

FIGURE 10.6: SONS AND DAUGHTERS ARE EQUAL

policy of the GOI in this and indeed did not advise newly-married women to use the oral pill. A long discussion took place about whether we would say that oral pill *can* be used in the first birth interval. The medical personnel said there was no counter-

indication. Others said that if the GOI does not include this, we should follow the government's policies. Also, what if women indeed do not become pregnant after the use of the oral pill? They will blame the oral pill and it will have all kinds of consequences for women if they do not get a child (remarriage of their husband, separation). The Dutch shared their experience that in the Netherlands every woman can use the oral pill, including women who do not have children. Keeping in mind the concept of informed choice, we finally decided to include information that the oral pill can be used by all women, even those who are newly wed. Only later did we learn that the GOI had altered its policy and now recommends the oral pill for women who do not have a child yet.

10.2.6 PRE-TESTING AND SENSITIZATION

All the scripts and pictures were pre-tested in order to get feedback from the villagers. The villagers made several remarks on the first version of the cards. One example concerned menstruation cloths which had to be dried in a hygienic way. To depict unhygienic circumstances, the card depicts cloths drying on a wood stack with cowdung and some insects. As it was necessary to bring attention to the insects, these were depicted somewhat big in size. During the field testing, a woman remarked that in the village 'we do not have such big animals in the wood stack!' Similarly, depicting small children turned out to be extremely difficult, because it is important that the age of the child matches the accompanying story. In addition, while focusing on close spacing, which—as respondents themselves indicated—makes women worn out, tired and look old (Chapter 6), it turned out to be difficult to depict women as weak and tired picture. However, we were pleased with the final product which conveys the emotions and feelings (Chapter 9) of women, men and children.

After pre-testing, the cards and scripts were finalized and printed.

Before starting the implementation, sensitization about Spandana was inititated: important people in the village, for

example village leaders, panchayat members, and Mahila Mandals were visited and the objectives of Spandana explained.

10.2.7 CHANGE AGENTS

The main change agents, namely people implementing the materials in the villages, were community workers and supervising community organizers. Both workers and organizers live in the villages and work in either their own or adjacent village(s). Because Spandana is a community-based intervention (see above), workers from the villages themselves were thought to be more able to relate to practices and perceptions of people in the village. Moreover, as Spandana aims to provide educational sessions at timings convenient for the villagers, which is commonly at the night, community workers and organizers had to be from the villages themselves. Most workers and organizers are young, some are married, some unmarried. Most of them are female while a smaller number are male. The male volunteers cannot address all topics, for example information on a sensitive topic as white discharge. The workers and organizers are supervised by two field coordinators and a campaign officer.

10.2.8 EDUCATIONAL GROUP SESSIONS AND MONITORING

Educational sessions, using flashcards and accompanying scripts, are conducted by the workers and organizers at night. Before implementation, an additional baseline survey was conducted in the 54 villages in Dharwad *taluka*. Community workers and organizers made maps of their villages and collected data on each household and each member of the household (name, age, education, marital status, pregnancy/delivery status, etc). This baseline is updated every year. The main objective of this survey is to identify the risk and target groups, to monitor the progress of Spandana, and to make evaluation at a later stage feasible. Based on the baseline survey, groups are identified in the villages among whom the materials are distributed. Monitoring of activities (group sessions, supportive activities) is included in Spandana and conducted by the researchers from PRC Dharwad.

10.2.9 COGNITIVE AND EMOTIONAL MESSAGES: SUPPORTIVE ACTIVITIES

Besides the so-called cognitive messages, i.e. focusing on acquirement of knowledge and information, Spandana also conducts so-called supportive activities. An important activity is for example the food demonstration. In the flashcards about anaemia and *hasi may* during menarche, emphasis is put on proper nutrition and the need to include food from all five nutritional groups. Rather than only conveying the message, demonstrations are organized to show how a balanced diet can be achieved. Spandana's coordinators show how to prepare a special dish with local food items (*tali pett*) including food from all five nutritional groups and especially green vegetables.

Two more supportive activities which employ research findings are organized in Spandana: singing *soobhana* and the felicitation of pregnant women (*udi tumbuvudu*). As the research revealed (Chapter 9), almost every event in the reproductive career (menarche, marriage, the first pregnancy) is celebrated with a ceremony and *soobhanas*. In Spandana, singers of *soobhana* are invited in a special function to sing special songs. In the *soobhana* on menarche, for example (Chapter 9), references are made to food provided to the girl who has reached maturity. Texts of *soobhanas* can be slightly changed or adapted, conveying a specific message, in this case, to add some green vegetables to the diet of young girls.

In addition, the research pointed out (Chapter 9) that every ceremony in the reproductive career is accompanied by the custom of *udi tumbuvudu*, filling the *udi*. One of these ceremonies is the *kubasa* during first pregnancy, which is commonly celebrated within the family, within the private domain. Spandana organizes special meetings for women who are pregnant for the first time in an important place in the village, for example, a temple or the *panchayat* building. Thus, pregnant women and their related health problems during pregnancy and delivery are situated in the public domain rather than only in the private domain. For example, emphasizing the responsibility of the community rather than only the individual family to take care of Safe Motherhood issues, e.g. providing transport in case of

emergencies. During these public meetings, relevant flashcards of Spandana are presented, namely those cards related to pregnancy, delivery, development of the foetus and food intake. Then, the pregnant women are felicitated by filling their *udi* (betel nut and leaves, banana, some grains, and a blouse piece) and *soobhanas*.

10.3 Summary and Discussion

In this chapter, we have described how the research results were translated into a reproductive health intervention. As mentioned above, Spandana is a culturally relevant intervention, based on the assumption that people will easily relate to and absorb information that takes into account their way of thinking. Whether Spandana has been successful in this approach will be ascertained in the near future when impacts on attitudes and knowledge will be measured. Interventions taking into account cultural aspects are necessarily limited to a certain area and region. At the moment on-going discussions pertain to upscaling the intervention to other groups in Dharwad *taluka*, e.g. urban slums or villages in the economically poorer parts of Karnataka.

The present research was a long-term research: the fieldwork started in 1996 and the initial results were released in March 2000, only after which Spandana could be launched. At present, we apply more rapid research methods, such as Focus Group Discussions, in order to be able to translate research into educational material more quickly.

Researchers and NGOs working together sounds easy, but it is actually a difficult undertaking, as the objectives of the involved parties differ. A pertinent issue concerns responsibility: would the primary responsibility to link research and intervention fall on the researchers or the NGOs? Our view is that researchers have, besides a scientific responsibility to publish their research, a moral responsibility to ensure that research conducted among poor people actually returns to those in need. And those who would benefit from the research findings.

References

Aziz, K.M.A. and C. Maloney (1985), 'Life Stages, Gender and Fertility in Bangladesh', Dhaka: International Centre for Diarrhoeal Disease Research, Bangladesh, Monographs Series 3.

Ajzen, I. and M. Fishbein (1980), *Understanding Attitudes and Predicting Social Behaviour*, Prentice-Hall, Englewood Cliffs, New York.

Ajzen, I. (1991), 'The Theory of Planned Behaviour', *Organisational Behaviour and Human Decision Processes*, 50, pp. 179-211.

Baird, D.D. et al. (1993), 'The Relationship between Reduced Fecundability and Subsequent Foetal Loss', in R. Gray, H. Leridon and A. Spira (eds.), *Biomedical and Demographic Determinants of Reproduction*, Clarendon Press, Oxford, pp. 329-44.

Bandura, A. (1982), 'Self-efficacy Mechanism in Human Agency', *American Psychologist*, 37(2), pp. 22-147.

——, (1986), *Social Foundations of Thought and Action: A Social Cognitive Theory*, Prentice-Hall, Englewood Cliffs, N.J.

Basu, A.M. (1989b), 'Is Discrimination in Food Really Necessary for Explaining Sex Differentials in Childhood Mortality?' *Population Studies*, 43, pp. 193-210.

Becker, S. (1993), 'The Determinants of Adolescent Fertility with Special Reference to Biological Variables', in R. Gray, H. Leridon and A. Spira (eds.), *Biomedical and Demographic Determinants of Reproduction*, Clarendon Press, Oxford, pp. 21-49.

Bhargava, S.K., Singh, K.K. and B.N. Saxena (1991), ICMR Task Force National Collaborative Study on Identification of High Risk Families, Mothers and Outcome of Their Off-springs with Particular Reference to the Problem of Maternal Nutrition, Low Birth Weight, Perinatal and Infant Morbidity and Mortality in Rural and Urban Slum Communities, *Indian Pediatrics*, 28(12), pp. 1473-80.

Bhat, M.B. and R.L. Patil (1994), 'Human Development Indicators for Karnataka: A District Level Analysis Report', JSS College, Institute of Economic Research, Dharwad.

Bongaarts, J. and R.G. Potter (1983), 'Fertility, Biology and Behaviour. An Analysis of the Proximate Determinants', *Studies in Population*, Academic Press, New York.

Bongaarts, J. (1982), 'The Fertility Inhibiting Effects of the Intermediate Fertility Variables', *Studies in Family Planning*, 13, pp. 179-89.

Bosch, A.M. (2005), *Adolescents' Reproductive Health in Rural Bangladesh*, Rozenberg Publishers, Amsterdam.

Bruijn de, B.J. (1992), 'The Concept of Rationality in Social Sciences', PDOD-paper, no. 9, Amsterdam.

—— (1993), 'Interdisciplinary Backgrounds of Fertility Theory', PDOD-paper, no. 16, Amsterdam.

—— (1999), '*Foundations of Demographic Theory*: *Choice*, Process, *Context*', NethurD Publications, Thela Thesis, Amsterdam.

Caldwell, J. (1976), 'Toward a Restatement of Demographic Transition Theory', *Population and Development Review*, vol. 2, nos. 2-3, pp. 321-66.

Caldwell, J. (1982), *Theory of Fertility Decline*, Academic Press, London.

Cates, W., R.T. Rolfs and S.O. Aral (1993), 'The Pathophysiology and Epidemiology of Sexually Transmitted Diseases in Relation to Pelvic Inflammatory Disease and Infertility', in R. Gray, H. Leridon and A. Spira (eds.), *Biomedical and Demographic Determinants of Reproduction*, Clarendon Press, Oxford, pp. 101-25.

Chin, D. (1999), 'HIV-related Sexual Risk Assessment among Asian/Pacific Islander American Women: An Inductive Model'. *Social Science and Medicine*, 49, 2, pp. 241-51.

Coale and Trussel (1974), 'Model Fertility Schedules: Variations in the Age Structure of Child Bearing in Human Populations', *Population Index*, 40, pp. 195-258.

Coleman, J.S. (1990), *Foundations of Social Theory*, Belknap Press, Harvard University Press, Cambridge (Mass).

Cumming, D.C. (1993), 'The Effects of Excercise and Nutrition on the Menstrual Cycle', in R. Gray, H. Leridon and A. Spira (eds.), *Biomedical and Demographic Determinants of Reproduction*, Clarendon Press, Oxford, pp. 132-56.

D'Andrade, R.G. (1984), 'Cultural Meaning Systems', in R.A. Schweder and R.A. Levine (eds.), *Culture Theory: Essays on Mind, Self and Emotion*, Cambridge University Press, Cambridge, pp. 88-119.

—— (1992), 'Schemas and Motivation', in R.G. D'Andrade and C. Strauss (eds.), *Human Motives and Cultural Models*, Cambridge University Press, Cambridge, pp. 23-44.

—— (1995), *The Development of Cognitive Anthropology*, Cambridge University Press, Cambridge.

Davis, K. and J. Blake (1956), 'Social Structure and Fertility: An Analytical Framework', *Economic Development and Cultural Change*, 4(4), pp. 212-35.

DGIS (1994), 'Family Planning Reproductive Gezondheid in Ontwikkelings-Samenwerking' (Family Planning and Reproductive Health in Development Cooperation), Dutch Ministry of Foreign Affairs, The Hague.

Dhanalakshmi, N. (1993), 'Demographic Correlates of Infant Mortality in Rural Areas', *Population Education News*, 20(4), pp. 21-3.

Dharmalingam, A. and S.P. Morgan (1996), 'Women's Work, Autonomy and Birth Control: Evidence from Two South Indian Villages', *Population Studies*, 50, pp. 187-201.

Denzau A.T. and D.C. North (1994), 'Shared Mental Models: Ideologies and Institutions', *Kyklos*, 47(1), pp. 3-31.

Draak, den M (2003), *Early Life Changes: Transition in Pregnancy and Birth Outcome in South India*, Rozenberg Publishers, Amsterdam.

Dubois, A.J.A. (1994), *Hindu Manners, Customs and Ceremonies*, 3rd edn., Rupa, New Delhi.

Dyson, T. and M. Moore (1983), 'On Kinship Structure, Female Autonomy and Demographic Behaviour in India', *Population and Development Review* 9 (1), pp. 35-60.

Ford, K. and S.L. Huffmann (1993), 'Maternal Nutrition, Infant Feeding, and Post-Partum Amenorrhoea: Recent Evidence from Bangladesh', in R. Gray, H. Leridon and A. Spira (eds.), *Biomedical and Demographic Determinants of Reproduction*, Clarendon Press, Oxford, pp. 383-90.

Ford, K. and Y.J. Kim (1993), 'Demographic Research on Lactational Amenorrhoea', in R. Gray, H. Leridon and A. Spira (eds.), *Biomedical and Demographic Determinants of Reproduction* Clarendon Press, Oxford, pp. 359-71.

Foster, A. J. Menken, A.K.M.A. Chowdhury and J. Trussel (1986), 'Female Reproductive Development: a Hazards Model Analysis', *Social Biology*, 33(3-4), pp. 183-99.

Frawley, D. (1989), '*Ayurvedic Healing: A Comprehensive Guide*', Motilal Banarsidass, New Delhi.

Gopalan, C. (1989), 'Women and Nutrition in India—General Considerations', in C. Gopalan and S. Kaur (eds.), *Women and Nutrition in India*, Nutrition Foundation of India, New Delhi, pp. 1-16.

Gray, R., H. Leridon and A. Spira (eds.) (1993), *Biomedical and Demographic Determinants of Reproduction* Clarendon Press, Oxford.

Greenhalgh S. (1989), *New Directions in Fertility Research: Anthropological Perspectives*, International Population Conference, IUSSP, New Delhi, vol. 3, pp. 437-49.

—— (1994), 'Anthropological Contributions to Fertility Theory', Working Paper no. 64. Population Council, New York.

—— (1995), *Situating Fertility: Anthropology and Demography Ingenuity*, Cambridge University Press, Cambridge.

Gujral, S., A. Chohan and T. Gopaldas (1992), 'Age and Sex-wise Child Mortality and the Influencing Socio-Economic Factors in a Rural and Tribal Population in Western India', *Indian Journal of Maternal and Child Health*, 3(4), pp. 113-17.

Haandrikman, K. (2000), *Coping with Time: Measurement and Perceptions of Age and Duration in Reproductive Health Surveys*, Population Research Centre, University of Groningen, The Netherlands.

Harkness, S., C.M. Super and C.H. Keefer (1992), 'Learning to be an American Parent: How Cultural Models Gain Directive Force', in R.G. D'Andrade and C. Strauss (eds.), *Human Motives and Cultural Models*, Cambridge University Press, Cambridge, pp. 163-78.

Harris, M. (1975), *Cultural People, Nature: An Introduction to General Anthropology*, Harper and Row Publishers, New York.

Hobcraft, J., J.W. McDonald and S.O. Rutstein (1985), 'Demographic Determinants of Infant and Early Child Mortality: a Comparative Analysis', *Population Studies*, 39, pp. 363-85.

Holland, D.C. (1992), 'How Cultural Systems Become Desire: A Case Study of American Romance', in R.G. D'Andrade and C. Strauss (eds.) *Human Motives and Cultural Models*, Cambridge University Press, Cambridge, pp. 61-89.

Hutter, I. (1994), *Being Pregnant in South India: Nutrition of Women and Well-being of Children*, Thesis Publisher, Amsterdam.

Hutter, I., et al. (1996), 'Fertility Change in India', RIVM Report, RIVM, Bilthoven.

Hutter, I. (1998), 'Reproductive Health and Child Spacing in Rural South India: Background Report to the Project', *Demographic Reports* 23, Population Research Centre, University of Groningen, The Netherlands.

Hutter, I. et al. (1999), 'Reproductive Health and Child Spacing in Rural South India: Survey Basis Report', *Demographic Reports* 26, Population Research Centre, University of Groningen, The Netherlands.

Hutter, I. et al. (2002), 'Reproductive Health and Child Spacing in rural South India: Basic Report In-depth Interviews, Female and Male Perspective', *Demographic Reports* 27, Population Research Centre, University of Groningen, The Netherlands.

Isaacs, S. and Fincancioglu, N. (1989), 'Promoting Family-Planning for Better Health: Policies and Programme Implications', *Population Bulletin*, United Nations, 26, pp. 102-25.

IPPF (1993), 'Meeting Challenges: Promoting Choices: A Report on the 40th Anniversary IPPF Family Planning Congres', New Delhi and IPPF, London.

Islam, M.M. and H.T.A. Khan (1993), 'Pattern of Coital Frequency in Rural Bangladesh', *Journal of Family Welfare*, 39(2), pp. 38-43.

Jager, M. de (1997), 'Reproductive Health: Proximate Determinants and Outcomes of an Integrated Model: A Case Study of the State of Karnataka, India', Population Research Centre, University of Groningen, The Netherlands.

James, W.P.T., A. Ferro-Luzi, and J.C. Waterlow (1988), 'Definition of Chronic Deficiency in Adults. Report of a Working Group Party of the International Dietary Energy Consultative Group', *European Journal of Clinical Nutrition* 42, pp. 969-82.

Jansen, R.P. (1984), 'Fertility in Older Women', *IPPF Medical Bulletin* 18(2), pp. 4-6.

Janssen, F. (2000), *Birth Intervals and Images on Childhood in Rural South India*, Population Research Centre, University of Groningen, The Netherlands.

Jeyaseelan, L. and B. Antoniswamy (1992), 'Pattern of Menstrual Cycle Length in South Indian Women: A Prospective Study', *Social Biology* 39(3-4), pp. 306-9.

Kakar, S. (1989), *Intimate Relations: Exploring Indian Sexuality*, Penguin Books, Delhi.

Knodel, J. (1978), 'Natural Fertility in Preindustrial Germany', *Population Studies* 32, pp. 481-510.

Koenig, M.A. and G.H.C. Foo (1992), 'Patriarchy, Women's Status, and Reproductive Behaviour in Rural North India', *Demography India*, 21(2), pp. 145-66.

Kost, K. and S. Amin (1992), Reproductive and Socio-economic Determinants of Child Survival: Confounded, Interactive, and Age-dependent Effects', *Social Biology* 39(12), pp. 139-50.

Kusin, J.A., Sri Kardjati and U.H. Renqvist (1992), 'Maternal Body Mass Index: The Functional Significance during Reproduction', Paper prepared for the Workshop on the Functional Significance of Low Body Mass Index, November 1992, Rome.

Kusin, J.A., Sri Kardjati, U.H. Renqvist and K.Goei (1994a), 'Reproduction and Maternal Nutrition in Madura, Indonesia', *Tropical and Geographical Medicine* 44, pp. 248-55.

Kusin, J.A., Sri Kardjati and U.H. Renquist (1994b), 'Chronic Undernutrition among Women of Reproductive Age', in J.A. Kusin and Sri Kardjati (eds.), *Maternal and Child Nutrition in Madura, Indonesia*, Royal Tropical Institute, Amsterdam, pp. 125-48.

Kusum (1983), 'Low Birth Weight, Maternal Nutrition and Birth Spacing', *Assignment Children*, 61/63, pp. 177-91.

Lad, V. (1992), *Ayurveda, de leer der zelfgenezing* ['Ayurveda, the Approach of Self Medication (in Dutch)], Amsterdam: Uitgeverij Schors.

Leridon, H. (1993), 'Fecundability and Postpartum Sterility: An Insuperable Interaction?', in R. Gray, H. Leridon and A. Spira (eds.), *Biomedical and Demographic Determinants of Reproduction*, Clarendon Press, Oxford, pp. 346-58.

Lindenberg, S.M. (1990), 'Towards the Construction of Interdisciplinary Theoretical Models to Explain Demographic Behaviour; a Comment', in C.A. Hazeu and G.A.B. Frinking, (eds.), *Emerging Issues in*

Demographic Research, Elseviers Science Publishers, Amsterdam, pp. 199-217.

Malhotra, A., R. Vanneman and S. Kishor (1995), 'Fertility, Dimensions of Patriarchy, and Development in India', *Population and Development Review* 21(2), pp. 281-25.

Maslow, A.H. (1970), *Motivation and Personality* 2nd edn., Harper and Row, New York.

Mauldin, W.P. and J.A. Ross (1994), 'Prospects and Programs for Fertility Reduction 1990-2015', *Studies in Family Planning* 25, pp. 77-110.

McNeilly, A.S. (1993), 'Breastfeeding and Fertility', in R. Gray, H. Leridon and A. Spira (eds.), *Biomedical and Demographic Determinants of Reproduction*, Clarendon Press, Oxford, pp. 391-412.

McNicoll, G. (1985), 'The Nature of Institutional and Community Effects on Demographic Behaviour: A Discussion', in J.B. Casterline (ed.), *The Collection and Analysis of Community Data*, International Statistical Institute, Voorburg, pp. 177-84.

—— (1989), *Concepts and Framework Needed for a Better Understanding of Socio-demographic Processes*, International Population Conference, IUSSP, New Delhi, vol. 3, pp. 423-36.

—— (1994), 'Institutional Analysis of Fertility', Working Paper no. 62, Population Council, New York.

Meredith, J.A. (1993), 'Statistical Evidence of Links between Maternal Nutrition and Post-partum Infertility', in R. Gray, H. Leridon and A. Spira (eds.), *Biomedical and Demographic Determinants of Reproduction*, Clarendon Press, Oxford, pp. 372-82.

Ministry of Health and Family Welfare (1991), *Family Welfare Yearbook 1990-1991*, New Delhi.

—— (1992), *Action Plan for Revamping the Family Welfare Programme in India*, New Delhi.

Nag, M. (1982), *Modernization and its Impact on Fertility: The Indian Scene*, Centre for Policy Studies, Working Papers no. 84, The Population Council, New York.

Nair, N. (1983), 'On a Distribution of First Conception Delays in the Presence of Adolescent Fertility', *Demography India* 12(2), pp. 269-75.

Nath, D.C., K.C. Land and K.K. Singh (1994), 'Birth Spacing, Breastfeeding, and Early Child Mortality in a Traditional Indian Society: A Hazards Model Analysis', *Social Biology* 41(3-4), pp. 168-80

North, D.C. (1994), 'Economic Performance Through Time', *American Economic Review* 84(3), pp. 359-68.

Oppenheim Mason, K. (1995a), *Gender and Demographic Change: What do we Know*? IUSSP, Liege.

—— (1995b), 'Is the Situation of Women in Asis Improving or Deteriorating?', *Asia-Pacific Population Research Reports* 6.

Population Reference Bureau (1986), 'Family Planning Saves Lives: A Strategy for Maternal and Child Survival', IMPACT Project, Population Reference Bureau, Washington D.C.

Quinn, N. (1997), 'Research on Shared Task Solution', in C. Strauss and N. Quinn (eds.), *A Cognitive Theory of Cultural Meaning*, Cambridge University Press, Cambridge, pp. 137-88.

Rahman, O. and J. Menken (1993), 'Age at Menopause and Fecundity Presiding Menopause', in R. Gray, H. Leridon and A. Spira (eds.), *Biomedical and Demographic Determinants of Reproduction*, Clarendon Press, Oxford, pp. 65-84.

Raina, B.L. (1994), *The Population Challenge*, B.R. Publishing Corporation, Delhi.

Rajeswari, N.V. and I. Hutter (1998), 'Reproductive Health and Child Spacing in Rural South India', Census basic report, *Demographic Reports 25*, Population Research Centre, University of Groningen, The Netherlands.

Rees (1995), 'The Age of Menarche', *Orgyn* 4, pp. 2-4.

Riley, A.P., J.L. Samuelson and S.L. Huffman (1993), 'The Relationship of Age at Menarche and Fertility in Undernourished Adolescents', in R. Gray, H. Leridon and A. Spira (eds.), *Biomedical and Demographic Determinants of Reproduction*, Clarendon Press, Oxford, pp. 50-64.

Rokeach, M. (1973), *The Nature of Human Values*, New York: Free Press.

Rodriguez G. and R. Aravena (1991), Socio-economic Factors and the Transition to Low Fertility in Less Developed Countries, a Comparative Analysis', in Demographic and Health Surveys World Conference, Columbia Md. 1, pp. 39-72.

Runyan, W.M. (1984), *Life Histories and Psychobiography: Explorations in Theory and Method*, Oxford University Press, New York.

Simon, H. (1986), 'Rationality in Psychology and Economics', in R.B. Hogarth and M.W. Reder (eds.), *Rational Choice: The Contrast Between Economics and Pyschology*, University of Chicago Press, Chicago, pp. 25-40.

Simpson, J.E. and S. Carson (1993), 'Biological Causes of Foetal Loss', in R. Gray, H. Leridon and A. Spira (eds.), *Biomedical and Demographic Determinants of Reproduction*, Clarendon Press, Oxford, pp. 297-315.

Singh, K.K. et al. (1993), 'Analysis of birth intervals in India's Uttar Pradesh and Kerala States', *Journal of Biosocial Sciences* 25 (2), pp. 143-53.

Singh, S. and D. Wulf (1994), 'Estimated Levels of Induced Abortion in Six Latin American Countries', *International Family Planning Perspectives* 20, pp. 4-13.

Smith, H.L. (1989), 'Integrating Theory and Research on the Institutional

Determinants of Fertility', *Demography* 26(2), pp. 171-84.
Srinivas, M.N. (1976), *The Remembered Village*, Berkely, Los Angeles, London: University of California Press.
Strauss, A. and J. Corbin (eds.) (1997), *Grounded Theory in Practice*, Sage Publications, Thousand Oaks, California.
Strauss, A. and J. Corbin (1998), *Basics of Qualitative Research: Techniques and Procedures for Developing Grounded Theory*, Sage Publications, Thousand Oaks, California.
Strauss, C. (1992), 'Models and Motives', in R.G. D'Andrade and C. Strauss (eds.) *Human Motives and Cultural Models*, Cambridge University Press, Cambridge, pp. 1-20.
Sujatha, D.S. and M.S.R. Murthy (1993), 'Husband–Wife Communication and Fertility among Two Sects of Brahmins', *Journal of Family Welfare* 39(4), pp. 26-30.
Spira, A. et al. (1993), 'Conception Probability and Pregnancy Outcome in Relation to Age, Cycle Regularity and Timing of Intercourse', in R. Gray, H. Leridon and A. Spira (eds.), *Biomedical and Demographic Determinants of Reproduction*, Clarendon Press, Oxford, pp. 271-84.
Udry, J.R. (1993), 'Coitus as Demographic Behaviour', in R. Gray, H. Leridon and A. Spira (eds.), *Biomedical and Demographic Determinants of Reproduction*, Clarendon Press, Oxford, pp. 85-97.
UNICEF (1991), 'Children and Women in India: A Situation Analysis, 1990', UNICEF, New Delhi.
Vianen van, H.A.W. et al. (1994), 'Fertility Change: A Global Integrated Perspective' RIVM Report, Bilthoven.
Weinstein, M., J. Wood and C. Ming-Cheng (1993), 'Age Patterns of Fecundability', in R. Gray, H. Leridon and A. Spira (eds.), *Biomedical and Demographic Determinants of Reproduction*, Clarendon Press, Oxford, pp. 209-27.
Westoff, C.F., L. Bumpass and N.B. Ryder (1969), 'Oral Contraception, Coital Frequency and Time Required to Conceive', *Social Biology*, 16, pp. 1-10.
Wilcox, A.J. et al. (1993), 'Endocrine Detection of Conception and Early Foetal Loss', in R. Gray, H. Leridon and A. Spira (eds.), *Biomedical and Demographic Determinants of Reproduction*, Clarendon Press, Oxford, pp. 317-28.
Willekens, F.J. (1989), 'Understanding the Interdependence Between Parallel Careers', Paper Presented at the Workshop on Female Labour Market Behaviour and Fertility: Preferences, Restrictions and Behaviour, NIDI, The Hague.
—— (1990), 'Beweging in de demografie' ('Movement in Demography') (Oratie), Rijksuniversiteit Groningen (in Dutch).
—— (1992), 'Models of Man in Demography', in H.A. Becker (ed.),

Dynamics of Cohort and Generations Research, Thesis Publishers, Amsterdam, pp. 253-81.

World Health Organization (WHO) (1984), 'Health and Family Planning', *In Point of Fact*, vol. 23, WHO, Geneva, pp. 1-4.

—— (1991), *Maternal Mortality: A Global Fact Book*, WHO, Geneva.

Index